I0767465

# THE MIND DIET FOR CARDIOVASCULAR WELLNESS

A comprehensive guide to nourishing your heart and enhancing cardiovascular health with expert tips ad 150+ delicious mind diet recipes

TERESA MILLER

# COPYRIGHT ©
### *All rights reserved.*

No part of this book may be reproduced in any form or by any electronic or mechanical means, including information storage and retrieval systems, without permission in writing from the publisher, except by a reviewer who may quote brief passages in a review.

The information contained in this book is based on the author's research and experience. While the author has made every effort to provide accurate and up-to-date information, errors and omissions may occur. The author and publisher assume no responsibility for any errors or omissions or for any actions taken based on the information contained in this book.

The information contained in this book is provided "as is," without warranty of any kind, express or implied, including but not limited to the warranties of merchantability, fitness for a particular purpose, or non-infringement. In no event shall the author or publisher be liable for any claim, damages, or other liability, whether in an action of contract, tort, or otherwise, arising from, out of, or in connection with the book or the use or other dealings in the book.

# TABLE OF CONTENTS

# CHAPTER THREE----------------------------------------------165

## DESSERT RECIPES----------------------------------------------165

# CONCLUSION ----------------------------------------------211

# INTRODUCTION

In the intricate symphony of our well-being, few instruments play as crucial a role as the heart. Often described as the rhythmic maestro of our bodies, the heart tirelessly pumps life-sustaining blood, ensuring the vitality of every cell, every organ, and every thought that fuels our existence. Yet, in the modern whirlwind of fast-paced lifestyles and dietary complexities, our hearts endure unprecedented challenges, facing the looming threat of heart disease.

Heart disease stands as a formidable adversary, casting a shadow over millions worldwide. According to the World Health Organization, cardiovascular diseases claim more lives annually than any other ailment, underscoring the urgency of prioritizing heart health.

However, in this landscape of concern, hope emerges from the synthesis of scientific discovery and dietary wisdom. Enter the MIND diet—a nutritional regimen meticulously crafted to nourish not just the body but specifically the mind and the heart. The Mediterranean-DASH Intervention for Neurodegenerative Delay (MIND) diet isn't just another dietary regimen; it's a symphony of carefully selected foods designed to protect cognitive function and, significantly, fortify the heart against the ravages of cardiovascular disease.

At the epicenter of our vitality lies the heart, an organ that tirelessly fuels our existence. Its ceaseless rhythm orchestrates our every breath, every step, and every moment. Yet, despite its pivotal role, the heart confronts an array of adversaries, from sedentary lifestyles and stress to poor dietary choices and genetic predispositions. Heart health isn't just a matter of physical wellness; it's the cornerstone of our ability to live, love, and thrive.

Amidst this challenge, the MIND diet emerges as a beacon of promise—a dietary approach tailored not just for physical health but specifically for the protection and nourishment of our most vital muscle, the heart. By synthesizing the best of the Mediterranean and DASH diets, the MIND diet champions the inclusion of brain-boosting foods that incidentally confer immeasurable benefits upon the heart.

Through meticulous research and scientific backing, the MIND diet showcases a synergistic blend of fruits, vegetables, whole grains, nuts, and lean proteins, each playing a pivotal role in fortifying cardiovascular health. Its emphasis on berries rich in antioxidants, leafy greens teeming with nutrients, and the omega-3 fatty acids abundant in fish presents a palette of culinary delights that safeguard not just cognitive sharpness but also shield the heart from the perils of cardiovascular disease.

In this comprehensive guide, we embark on a journey—a journey that transcends the conventional boundaries of diet and delves into the intricacies of heart health. We unravel the mysteries of the MIND diet, exploring its nuances, delving into scientific insights, and equipping you with the knowledge and tools to not just nourish your mind but also fortify your heart against the tides of heart disease.

Join us in this odyssey towards optimal heart health through the prism of the MIND diet—a journey that doesn't just promise longevity but empowers you to embrace life with vitality and vigor.

# CHAPTER ONE

## THE CORE PRINCIPLES OF THE MIND DIET

The MIND diet, short for Mediterranean-DASH Intervention for Neurodegenerative Delay, is a dietary pattern specifically designed to support brain health and reduce the risk of cognitive decline. It combines elements from two well-known diets: the Mediterranean diet and the DASH (Dietary Approaches to Stop Hypertension) diet. While initially intended to enhance cognitive function and reduce the risk of neurodegenerative diseases like Alzheimer's, research has shown its potential benefits for heart health as well. The core principles of the MIND diet emphasize specific food groups and nutrients known to promote heart health:

Emphasis on Plant-Based Foods:

• Encourages a diet rich in vegetables, especially leafy greens like kale, spinach, and broccoli, which are high in vitamins, minerals, and antioxidants.

• Advocates for regular consumption of fruits, particularly berries like strawberries, blueberries, and raspberries, known for their potent antioxidants that benefit heart health.

Inclusion of Whole Grains:

• Supports the consumption of whole grains such as brown rice, quinoa, oats, and whole wheat, which are high in fiber and essential nutrients linked to heart health.

## Healthy Fats:

• Promotes the intake of healthy fats found in sources like olive oil, nuts (especially walnuts), seeds, and fatty fish (like salmon), which are abundant in omega-3 fatty acids associated with reducing the risk of heart disease and inflammation.

## Limiting Unhealthy Foods:

• Suggests limiting the intake of red meat, processed foods, sweets, and fried foods, which are associated with increased heart disease risk factors such as high cholesterol and inflammation.

## Moderation in Alcohol Consumption:

• Allows moderate intake of wine, particularly red wine, due to its potential heart-protective properties when consumed in moderation and as part of a balanced diet.

## DASH and Mediterranean Diet Fusion:

• Integrates aspects from both the DASH and Mediterranean diets, combining the emphasis on fruits, vegetables, whole grains, and healthy fats while also considering the impact of specific foods on heart health.

By following the MIND diet's core principles, individuals can adopt a dietary pattern that not only supports brain health and cognitive function but also potentially reduces the risk of heart disease. The focus on nutrient-dense, heart-healthy foods while limiting less beneficial options forms the cornerstone of the MIND diet's impact on cardiovascular wellness.

## THE ORIGIN OF THE MIND DIET

The MIND diet was developed based on research conducted by nutritional epidemiologists at Rush University Medical Center in Chicago. This dietary pattern originated from a study known as the "Rush Memory and Aging Project" (MAP) led by Dr. Martha Clare Morris, a nutritional epidemiologist, and her team.

The primary aim of the Rush Memory and Aging Project was to investigate lifestyle factors, particularly diet, and their impact on age-related cognitive decline and the risk of developing Alzheimer's disease and other forms of dementia.

Dr. Morris and her colleagues observed that certain dietary patterns, particularly those resembling the Mediterranean and DASH diets, showed promising effects on cognitive health. The Mediterranean diet emphasizes high consumption of fruits, vegetables, whole grains, healthy fats (such as olive oil), and moderate intake of fish and wine. The DASH diet (Dietary Approaches to Stop Hypertension) focuses on lowering high blood pressure by encouraging the consumption of fruits, vegetables, whole grains, lean proteins, and limiting sodium intake.

Combining key elements from these two diets, Dr. Morris and her team identified specific foods and nutrients associated with better brain health and reduced risk of cognitive decline. They then formulated the MIND diet, which stands for Mediterranean-DASH Intervention for Neurodegenerative Delay, as a modified dietary pattern that specifically targets brain health and aims to delay cognitive decline and reduce the risk of neurodegenerative diseases like Alzheimer's.

The MIND diet's distinctiveness lies in its focus on incorporating foods and nutrients that have been scientifically linked to better cognitive function, while also considering their potential benefits for overall health, including heart health. Over the years, research has supported the efficacy of the MIND diet in not only preserving cognitive abilities but also potentially reducing the risk of other age-related conditions, including cardiovascular diseases, by promoting a nutrient-rich and balanced eating pattern.

## HOW THE MIND DIET INTEGRATES ELEMENTS BENEFICIAL FOR HEART HEALTH

The MIND diet, primarily designed to support brain health and reduce the risk of cognitive decline, incorporates several elements that are also beneficial for heart health. While its core focus remains on cognitive function, the dietary principles of the MIND diet inadvertently promote cardiovascular wellness due to the inclusion of heart-healthy foods and nutrients.

Here's how the MIND diet integrates elements beneficial for heart health:

Emphasis on Plant-Based Foods:

• Vegetables: Leafy greens like kale, spinach, and broccoli are rich in vitamins, minerals, and antioxidants. These nutrients are known to support heart health by reducing inflammation and improving overall cardiovascular function.

• Berries: Blueberries, strawberries, and raspberries are high in antioxidants and flavonoids, which have been associated with a lower risk of heart disease by reducing oxidative stress and inflammation.

Whole Grains:

• Whole grains: Incorporating whole grains such as oats, brown rice, quinoa, and whole wheat provides fiber and essential nutrients. These help lower cholesterol levels and reduce the risk of heart disease and stroke.

Healthy Fats:

• Olive oil: A staple in the Mediterranean diet (a component of the MIND diet), olive oil contains monounsaturated fats that have been linked to improved heart health by reducing bad cholesterol levels.

• Nuts and Seeds: Walnuts, almonds, flaxseeds, and chia seeds are rich in omega-3 fatty acids, which have anti-inflammatory properties and can contribute to better heart health.

• Fatty Fish: Sources of omega-3s like salmon, mackerel, and trout are known to reduce the risk of heart disease and promote cardiovascular health.

Limiting Unhealthy Foods:

• Red Meat: The MIND diet advises limiting red meat consumption, which is often associated with an increased risk of heart disease when consumed excessively.

• Processed Foods and Sweets: Minimizing intake of processed foods and sweets helps reduce the intake of added sugars, trans fats, and unhealthy additives that can negatively impact heart health.

Moderate Alcohol Consumption:

• Moderate wine intake: The MIND diet suggests moderate consumption of wine, especially red wine, which contains antioxidants like resveratrol that may benefit heart health when consumed in moderation.

DASH and Mediterranean Diet Influence:

• By integrating elements from the DASH and Mediterranean diets, the MIND diet indirectly incorporates heart-healthy aspects such as lower sodium intake, balanced macronutrients, and a focus on nutrient-dense foods that support overall cardiovascular wellness.

The MIND diet's emphasis on nutrient-rich, plant-based foods, healthy fats, and the restriction of less healthy options aligns with dietary patterns linked to improved heart health. While originally designed for cognitive health, the MIND diet's composition inadvertently fosters a diet that supports a healthy heart, potentially reducing the risk of heart disease and contributing to overall cardiovascular well-being.

## WHAT IS HEART DISEASE?

Heart disease, also known as cardiovascular disease (CVD), refers to a group of conditions that affect the heart or blood vessels. It encompasses various disorders that can affect the heart's functionality, leading to complications ranging from mild to life-threatening. Some common types of heart disease include:

• Coronary Artery Disease (CAD): CAD is the most common type of heart disease. It occurs when the coronary arteries, responsible for supplying oxygen-rich blood to the heart muscle, become narrowed or blocked due to the buildup of plaque (atherosclerosis). This can lead to chest pain (angina), heart attacks, or myocardial infarctions.

• Heart Attack (Myocardial Infarction): A heart attack occurs when there's a sudden blockage in one of the coronary arteries, cutting off blood flow to a part of the heart. This deprivation of oxygen and nutrients can cause damage or death to the heart muscle cells.

• Heart Failure: Heart failure doesn't mean the heart has stopped working; rather, it refers to the heart's inability to pump blood effectively. It can happen gradually as the heart becomes weaker or suddenly after a heart attack or other heart-related conditions.

• Arrhythmias: These are irregular heartbeats that can manifest as tachycardia (rapid heartbeat), bradycardia (slow heartbeat), or other abnormal rhythms, potentially affecting the heart's ability to pump blood efficiently.

• Heart Valve Problems: Conditions affecting heart valves, such as stenosis (narrowing), regurgitation (leakage), or prolapse, can lead to disrupted blood flow through the heart.

• Congenital Heart Defects: These are structural problems present at birth, affecting the heart's structure and function. They can range from simple conditions to complex defects that require surgical intervention.

Prevention and Treatment:

Prevention strategies include adopting a healthy lifestyle with a balanced diet, regular exercise, not smoking, managing stress, and controlling conditions like high blood pressure, cholesterol, and diabetes. Treatment varies based on the type and severity of the heart condition and may involve medications, lifestyle changes, surgeries, or other interventions to manage symptoms and improve heart health. Regular medical check-ups and early intervention are crucial in preventing complications from heart disease.

# THE PREVALENCE OF HEART DISEASE

Heart disease is a prevalent health concern worldwide, impacting individuals of various ages, genders, and ethnicities. Its prevalence varies across regions and populations, but it remains a leading cause of morbidity and mortality globally.

Global Prevalence:

• High Prevalence: Heart disease, encompassing various cardiovascular conditions, is one of the most common health problems worldwide. It affects millions of people, contributing significantly to the global burden of disease.

• Mortality Rates: Heart disease, including coronary artery disease, heart attacks, and stroke, is a leading cause of death in many countries. It accounts for a significant percentage of deaths annually, contributing substantially to mortality rates worldwide.

• Geographical Variations: The prevalence of heart disease can differ significantly across regions. While it's prevalent in developed countries due to lifestyle factors, it's also increasingly becoming a concern in developing nations as lifestyles change, adopting more sedentary habits and unhealthy diets.

Several factors contribute to the prevalence of heart disease:

• Lifestyle Factors: Sedentary lifestyles, poor dietary habits high in saturated fats, cholesterol, and sodium, lack of physical activity, smoking, and excessive alcohol consumption contribute significantly to the development of heart disease.

• Age and Gender: The risk of heart disease increases with age, and men tend to have a higher risk at a younger age compared to women. However, after menopause, women's risk catches up due to hormonal changes.

• Genetic Predisposition: Family history of heart disease or genetic factors can increase an individual's susceptibility to developing heart-related conditions.

• Health Conditions: Conditions such as hypertension (high blood pressure), diabetes, obesity, and high cholesterol levels significantly elevate the risk of heart disease.

Impact on Healthcare:

• The prevalence of heart disease places a considerable burden on healthcare systems globally. Treatment, management, and interventions for heart-related conditions require significant healthcare resources, including medications, surgeries, cardiac procedures, and ongoing medical care.

- Efforts to reduce the prevalence of heart disease focus on public health initiatives, education about healthy lifestyle choices, promoting regular physical activity, advocating for a balanced diet, encouraging smoking cessation, managing stress, and increasing awareness about risk factors and preventive measures.

While the prevalence of heart disease remains a significant concern, preventive strategies and early interventions can help mitigate the risk and reduce its impact on individuals and healthcare systems, emphasizing the importance of adopting and maintaining a heart-healthy lifestyle. Regular screenings, early diagnosis, and proper management of risk factors play a vital role in preventing the onset and progression of heart-related conditions.

# THE RISK FACTORS ASSOCIATED WITH HEART DISEASE

Heart disease can develop due to a combination of various risk factors, both modifiable and non-modifiable, that contribute to the increased likelihood of cardiovascular problems. Understanding these risk factors is crucial in assessing and managing an individual's risk of developing heart-related conditions. Here are the primary risk factors associated with heart disease:

## Non-Modifiable Risk Factors:

• Age: The risk of heart disease increases with age. Men aged 45 and older and women aged 55 and older are at higher risk.

• Gender: Men generally have a higher risk of heart disease at a younger age, but post-menopausal women's risk becomes comparable to men due to hormonal changes.

• Family History: A family history of heart disease or a first-degree relative (parent or sibling) with early-onset heart disease can increase an individual's risk.

## Modifiable Risk Factors:

• High Blood Pressure (Hypertension): Elevated blood pressure forces the heart to work harder, increasing the risk of heart attack, stroke, and other heart-related complications.

• High Cholesterol Levels: Elevated levels of LDL ("bad") cholesterol and triglycerides contribute to the buildup of plaque in arteries, increasing the risk of atherosclerosis and heart disease.

• Smoking and Tobacco Use: Tobacco smoke damages blood vessels, increases blood pressure, reduces oxygen supply, and significantly raises the risk of heart disease.

• Diabetes: Poorly controlled diabetes increases the risk of heart disease, as high blood sugar levels can damage blood vessels and nerves that control the heart.

• Obesity and Physical Inactivity: Excess body weight, especially around the abdomen, coupled with a sedentary lifestyle, contributes to high blood pressure, high cholesterol, and an increased risk of heart disease.

• Unhealthy Diet: Diets high in saturated fats, trans fats, cholesterol, sodium, and refined sugars contribute to obesity, high cholesterol levels, hypertension, and increased risk of heart disease.

• Stress: Chronic stress can contribute to unhealthy behaviors like overeating, smoking, or alcohol abuse, affecting blood pressure and heart health.

• Excessive Alcohol Consumption: Consuming alcohol in excess can raise blood pressure, contribute to obesity, and increase the risk of heart disease.

Other Contributing Factors:

• Sleep Apnea: This sleep disorder is associated with an increased risk of hypertension, heart disease, and stroke.

• Poor Dental Health: Periodontal disease may be linked to an increased risk of heart disease.

• Certain Medications: Some medications, if not monitored or used properly, can contribute to heart-related complications.

Prevention and Management:

Understanding these risk factors is crucial for implementing preventive measures and lifestyle modifications. By adopting a heart-healthy lifestyle—such as a balanced diet, regular exercise, not smoking, managing stress, maintaining a healthy weight, and controlling underlying conditions like hypertension and diabetes—it's possible to significantly reduce the risk of developing heart disease and related complications. Regular medical check-ups and consultations with healthcare professionals can aid in assessing individual risks and developing personalized strategies for heart disease prevention and management.

# HOW DIET PLAYS A CRUCIAL ROLE IN PREVENTING HEART DISEASE.

Diet plays a pivotal role in preventing heart disease as it significantly influences several key risk factors associated with cardiovascular health. Making informed and healthy dietary choices can contribute to reducing the risk of developing heart-related conditions. Here are ways in which diet plays a crucial role in preventing heart disease:

Impact on Risk Factors:

• Controlling Cholesterol Levels: A diet high in saturated and trans fats contributes to elevated LDL ("bad") cholesterol levels, leading to plaque buildup in arteries. Choosing foods low in these unhealthy fats and incorporating sources of healthy fats, such as omega-3 fatty acids found in fish, nuts, and seeds, can help lower LDL cholesterol levels.

• Lowering Blood Pressure: Consuming a diet rich in fruits, vegetables, whole grains, and low-fat dairy products while reducing sodium intake can help manage blood pressure levels, reducing the risk of hypertension and heart disease.

• Managing Blood Sugar Levels: For individuals with diabetes or prediabetes, a balanced diet consisting of complex carbohydrates, lean proteins, and healthy fats helps manage blood sugar levels and reduces the risk of heart disease associated with diabetes.

• Reducing Inflammation: Certain foods high in antioxidants, such as fruits, vegetables, and whole grains, have anti-inflammatory properties that may reduce inflammation in the body, a factor linked to heart disease.

• Maintaining a Healthy Weight: A diet high in nutrient-dense, low-calorie foods like fruits, vegetables, and whole grains, combined with portion control and limiting high-calorie, processed foods, helps manage weight and reduces the risk of obesity — a significant risk factor for heart disease.

Specific Dietary Recommendations for Heart Health:

• Emphasis on Fruits and Vegetables: These are rich in vitamins, minerals, antioxidants, and fiber, all of which promote heart health.

• Whole Grains: Foods like brown rice, quinoa, oats, and whole wheat provide fiber and nutrients that support heart health by reducing cholesterol levels and improving blood vessel function.

• Healthy Fats: Incorporating sources of healthy fats like avocados, olive oil, nuts, and fatty fish (salmon, mackerel) can improve cholesterol levels and reduce the risk of heart disease.

• Limiting Saturated and Trans Fats: Reducing intake of foods high in saturated fats (found in fatty meats, full-fat dairy) and eliminating trans fats (found in processed foods) is crucial for heart health.

• Reducing Sodium: Lowering salt intake helps manage blood pressure, decreasing the risk of hypertension and heart disease.

Dietary Pattern Recommendations:

• Mediterranean Diet: This diet, rich in fruits, vegetables, whole grains, fish, nuts, and olive oil while limiting red meat and processed foods, is associated with a reduced risk of heart disease.

• DASH Diet: The Dietary Approaches to Stop Hypertension (DASH) diet, focusing on fruits, vegetables, lean proteins, and low-fat dairy while limiting sodium, can help manage blood pressure and reduce heart disease risk.

Lifestyle Integration:

Adopting a heart-healthy diet is just one aspect of overall heart disease prevention. Coupled with regular physical activity, stress management, maintaining a healthy weight, avoiding tobacco, and managing underlying health conditions, a balanced and nutritious diet significantly contributes to preventing heart disease and supporting overall cardiovascular wellness. Regular consultations with healthcare professionals and dietitians can help individuals develop personalized dietary plans tailored to their specific health needs and reduce their risk of heart disease.

The MIND diet emphasizes several key food groups that are not only beneficial for brain health (as the diet was initially designed for) but also contribute significantly to supporting heart health. These food groups are rich in nutrients, antioxidants, healthy fats, and fiber that are known to promote cardiovascular wellness. Here are the key food groups emphasized in the MIND diet that are particularly beneficial for heart health:

1. Vegetables:

• Leafy Greens: Kale, spinach, collard greens, and broccoli are packed with vitamins, minerals (such as potassium and magnesium), antioxidants (like vitamin C and beta-carotene), and dietary fiber. These nutrients support heart health by helping to regulate blood pressure, improve cholesterol levels, and reduce the risk of heart disease.

2. Berries:

• Blueberries, Strawberries, and Raspberries: These fruits are rich in antioxidants, such as flavonoids and anthocyanins, which have anti-inflammatory properties and help reduce oxidative stress. They contribute to improved heart health by potentially reducing the risk of cardiovascular diseases through their positive effects on blood vessel function and blood pressure regulation.

3. Whole Grains:

• Oats, Brown Rice, Quinoa, Whole Wheat: Whole grains are excellent sources of fiber, vitamins, minerals, and phytonutrients. Their consumption is associated with lower cholesterol levels, reduced risk of heart disease, and improved cardiovascular health due to their ability to lower blood pressure and support healthy blood vessel function.

4. Healthy Fats:

• Olive Oil: A staple in the Mediterranean diet (a component of the MIND diet), olive oil is rich in monounsaturated fats and antioxidants. It supports heart health by improving cholesterol levels and reducing inflammation.

• Nuts and Seeds: Almonds, walnuts, flaxseeds, chia seeds, and other nuts and seeds are high in omega-3 fatty acids, fiber, and plant-based proteins, all of which contribute to lowering LDL cholesterol, reducing inflammation, and supporting heart health.

5. Fatty Fish:

• Salmon, Mackerel, Trout: Fatty fish are excellent sources of omega-3 fatty acids, particularly EPA and DHA, which are associated with a decreased risk of heart disease. These fatty acids help reduce triglycerides, lower blood pressure, and prevent plaque buildup in arteries.

6. Other Heart-Healthy Foods:

• Legumes (Beans and Lentils): Legumes are high in protein, fiber, vitamins, and minerals while being low in fat. They support heart health by improving cholesterol levels and reducing the risk of heart disease.

Emphasizing these food groups as part of the MIND diet not only supports cognitive health but also contributes significantly to a heart-healthy eating pattern. By incorporating these nutrient-dense foods into regular meals, individuals following the MIND diet may benefit from improved cardiovascular wellness and reduced risk factors associated with heart disease.

The foods highlighted in the MIND diet are rich in various nutrients and compounds that contribute to heart health through several mechanisms. Here's a breakdown of the key nutrients and compounds within these foods that promote cardiovascular wellness:

1. Antioxidants:

• Found in Berries and Leafy Greens: Berries like blueberries, strawberries, and raspberries, as well as leafy greens such as kale and spinach, contain high levels of antioxidants like flavonoids, anthocyanins, and vitamin C. These antioxidants help reduce oxidative stress and inflammation in blood vessels, thereby supporting heart health by improving blood flow, reducing plaque formation, and protecting against cellular damage.

2. Omega-3 Fatty Acids:

• Present in Fatty Fish, Nuts, and Seeds: Fatty fish like salmon, mackerel, and trout, along with nuts (especially walnuts) and seeds (flaxseeds, chia seeds), contain omega-3 fatty acids, notably EPA (eicosapentaenoic acid) and DHA (docosahexaenoic acid). These fatty acids have anti-inflammatory properties, help lower triglycerides, reduce blood clotting, improve blood vessel function, and contribute to overall heart health by reducing the risk of heart disease and stroke.

3. Fiber:

• Abundant in Whole Grains, Fruits, Vegetables, and Legumes: Whole grains like oats, brown rice, quinoa, fruits, vegetables, and legumes (beans, lentils) are excellent sources of dietary fiber. Fiber helps lower LDL cholesterol levels, regulate blood sugar, improve digestive health, and aid in weight management, all of which are crucial factors in reducing the risk of heart disease and maintaining cardiovascular wellness.

4. Monounsaturated Fats and Polyphenols:

• Contained in Olive Oil: Olive oil is rich in monounsaturated fats and polyphenols, which have been associated with reducing LDL cholesterol levels, improving blood vessel function, and providing antioxidant and anti-inflammatory benefits that support heart health.

5. Plant Sterols and Phytonutrients:

• Found in Nuts, Seeds, and Whole Grains: Nuts, seeds, and whole grains contain plant sterols and phytonutrients, such as phytosterols and flavonoids, which contribute to lowering cholesterol levels, reducing inflammation, improving blood vessel function, and protecting against cardiovascular diseases.

6. Vitamins and Minerals:

• Present in Various Foods: Fruits, vegetables, nuts, seeds, and whole grains are rich in essential vitamins (like vitamin C, vitamin E) and minerals (such as potassium, magnesium) that play roles in reducing oxidative stress, maintaining healthy blood pressure, supporting proper heart muscle function, and overall heart health.

These nutrients and compounds work synergistically within the foods emphasized in the MIND diet, contributing to their collective impact on reducing heart disease risk factors and supporting optimal cardiovascular wellness when incorporated into a balanced and heart-healthy eating pattern.

## HOW THE MIND DIET SPECIFICALLY BENEFITS HEART HEALTH

The MIND diet, originally designed to support brain health and reduce the risk of cognitive decline, inadvertently offers several benefits that contribute significantly to heart health. While the primary focus remains on cognitive function, the dietary principles of the MIND diet incorporate foods and nutrients known to promote cardiovascular wellness. Here's how the MIND diet specifically benefits heart health:

• Rich in Fruits and Vegetables: The MIND diet places a strong emphasis on consuming a variety of colorful fruits and vegetables, such as berries, leafy greens, and other nutrient-dense produce. These foods are abundant in antioxidants, vitamins, minerals, and dietary fiber that support heart health by reducing inflammation, improving blood vessel function, and lowering the risk of heart disease.

• Inclusion of Whole Grains: Whole grains like oats, brown rice, and quinoa provide fiber, vitamins, and minerals that help lower cholesterol levels, regulate blood sugar, and contribute to overall heart health.

• Healthy Fats: Incorporating sources of healthy fats, such as olive oil, nuts, seeds, and fatty fish, provides essential omega-3 fatty acids and monounsaturated fats that help reduce LDL ("bad") cholesterol levels, lower triglycerides, and promote cardiovascular wellness.

Reduction of Risk Factors:

• Lowering LDL Cholesterol: The MIND diet's composition of foods like nuts, seeds, fruits, and vegetables that are rich in fiber, antioxidants, and healthy fats contributes to reducing LDL cholesterol levels, a significant risk factor for heart disease.

• Blood Pressure Management: By promoting foods high in potassium (such as leafy greens, fruits, and nuts) and low in sodium, the MIND diet supports healthy blood pressure levels, reducing the risk of hypertension and associated heart complications.

• Anti-Inflammatory Properties: The antioxidants and phytonutrients found in foods like berries, leafy greens, nuts, and olive oil have anti-inflammatory properties that help reduce inflammation in blood vessels, thereby promoting better heart health and reducing the risk of cardiovascular disease.

## Promotion of Overall Heart-Healthy Eating Pattern:

• Balanced Nutrient Intake: The MIND diet encourages a well-rounded intake of essential nutrients from a variety of food groups, which supports overall cardiovascular wellness.

• Stress Reduction: While not directly related to diet, the MIND diet's emphasis on overall lifestyle factors, including stress reduction techniques, indirectly contributes to heart health by helping manage stress, which is a risk factor for heart disease.

## Combination of Mediterranean and DASH Diet Principles:

• By integrating elements from the Mediterranean and DASH diets, the MIND diet combines the benefits of both patterns — such as emphasizing fruits, vegetables, whole grains, healthy fats, and lean proteins — contributing to a comprehensive approach to heart health.

In summary, the MIND diet, with its emphasis on heart-healthy foods, reduction of risk factors, promotion of a balanced eating pattern, and incorporation of anti-inflammatory and nutrient-rich foods, offers substantial benefits that support cardiovascular wellness and may potentially reduce the risk of heart disease when followed as part of a healthy lifestyle.

## SCIENTIFIC STUDIES AND EVIDENCE SUPPORTING THESE CLAIMS

Here are some general findings and areas of scientific research that support the relationship between the MIND diet and heart health.

• Observational Studies: Several observational studies have indicated a positive association between adherence to the MIND diet and a reduced risk of cardiovascular diseases. These studies have shown that a diet rich in fruits, vegetables, whole grains, nuts, and healthy fats—similar to the MIND diet—correlates with lower incidences of heart disease, reduced risk of hypertension, and better cardiovascular health outcomes.

• Antioxidants and Heart Health: Research has consistently shown that antioxidants present in foods like berries and leafy greens can help reduce oxidative stress and inflammation, which are critical factors in the development of heart disease. Antioxidants may contribute to improving endothelial function, reducing blood pressure, and supporting overall heart health.

• Omega-3 Fatty Acids: Numerous studies have demonstrated the beneficial effects of omega-3 fatty acids found in fatty fish, nuts, and seeds on heart health. These fats have been associated with reducing triglycerides, lowering the risk of arrhythmias, improving blood vessel function, and reducing the incidence of cardiovascular events.

• Whole Grains and Heart Health: Consumption of whole grains has been linked to a lower risk of heart disease. Studies suggest that the fiber, vitamins, minerals, and phytonutrients in whole grains contribute to improved cholesterol levels, reduced inflammation, and better cardiovascular outcomes.

• Mediterranean Diet and DASH Diet Influence: Research supporting the Mediterranean diet and DASH diet, from which the MIND diet draws its principles, has shown positive effects on heart health. These diets emphasize fruits, vegetables, whole grains, healthy fats, and lean proteins, contributing to reduced cardiovascular risk factors and better heart health outcomes.

While specific studies directly assessing the MIND diet's impact on heart health may be limited, the evidence supporting the individual components of the diet, such as fruits, vegetables, nuts, healthy fats, and whole grains, collectively contributes to the understanding of how adherence to a similar dietary pattern can positively influence cardiovascular wellness. Researchers continue to explore the comprehensive effects of the MIND diet on heart health, cognition, and overall well-being through ongoing studies and clinical trials.

# A COMPREHENSIVE LIST OF RECOMMENDED FOODS KNOWN TO IMPROVE HEART HEALTH

Here's a comprehensive list of recommended foods known to improve heart health:

1. Fruits:

• Berries: Blueberries, strawberries, raspberries, and blackberries are rich in antioxidants, fiber, and vitamins, supporting heart health.

• Citrus Fruits: Oranges, grapefruits, lemons, and limes are high in vitamin C, fiber, and flavonoids, which promote heart health.

2. Vegetables:

• Leafy Greens: Spinach, kale, Swiss chard, and collard greens are packed with vitamins, minerals, antioxidants, and fiber beneficial for heart health.

• Cruciferous Vegetables: Broccoli, cauliflower, Brussels sprouts, and cabbage contain antioxidants and fiber that support cardiovascular wellness.

3. Whole Grains:

• Oats: Rich in soluble fiber, oats help reduce LDL cholesterol levels and are beneficial for heart health.

• Brown Rice, Quinoa, Whole Wheat: Whole grains provide fiber, vitamins, and minerals that aid in lowering heart disease risk.

4. Fatty Fish:

• Salmon, Mackerel, Sardines, Trout: High in omega-3 fatty acids, these fish reduce inflammation, improve blood vessel function, and support heart health.

5. Nuts and Seeds:

• Almonds, Walnuts, Flaxseeds, Chia Seeds: Rich in omega-3 fatty acids, fiber, and antioxidants, nuts and seeds promote heart health when consumed in moderation.

6. Healthy Fats and Oils:

• Olive Oil: Contains monounsaturated fats and antioxidants, reducing LDL cholesterol and inflammation.

• Avocado: Packed with monounsaturated fats, fiber, and potassium, supporting heart health.

7. Legumes:

• Beans, Lentils, Chickpeas: High in fiber, protein, and antioxidants, legumes help lower cholesterol and manage blood sugar levels.

8. Low-Fat Dairy:

• Yogurt, Skim Milk: Provide calcium, potassium, and protein while being lower in saturated fats compared to whole-fat dairy options.

9. Herbs and Spices:

• Turmeric: Contains curcumin, which has anti-inflammatory properties beneficial for heart health.

• Garlic: Known to lower blood pressure and cholesterol levels, supporting cardiovascular wellness.

10. Dark Chocolate (in moderation):

• Contains Flavonoids: Dark chocolate with high cocoa content (70% or more) may have heart-protective benefits due to its flavonoid content.

11. Green Tea:

• Rich in Antioxidants: Contains catechins that may contribute to improved heart health and reduced risk of cardiovascular disease.

12. Red Wine (in moderation):

• Resveratrol: Found in red wine, resveratrol is an antioxidant associated with potential heart-protective effects when consumed in moderation as part of a balanced diet.

Incorporating these foods into a balanced diet, along with healthy lifestyle choices such as regular physical activity, not smoking, and managing stress, can significantly contribute to improved heart health and reduced risk of cardiovascular diseases.

## FOODS TO LIMIT OR AVOID DUE TO THEIR NEGATIVE IMPACT ON HEART HEALTH

To promote heart health, it's essential to limit or avoid certain foods that can have negative effects on cardiovascular wellness. Here's a list of foods to limit or avoid due to their potential negative impact on heart health:

1. Trans Fats:

• Partially Hydrogenated Oils: Found in many processed and packaged foods like baked goods, fried foods, margarine, and some spreads, trans fats raise LDL ("bad") cholesterol and lower HDL ("good") cholesterol, increasing the risk of heart disease.

2. Saturated Fats:

• High-Fat Meats: Fatty cuts of beef, pork, and lamb are high in saturated fats, which can raise LDL cholesterol levels.

• Full-Fat Dairy: Whole milk, cheese, butter, and cream contain saturated fats that can contribute to elevated cholesterol levels.

• Processed Meats: Bacon, sausage, hot dogs, and deli meats often contain saturated fats and high amounts of sodium, increasing the risk of heart disease.

3. Added Sugars:

• Sugary Beverages: Soda, sweetened juices, energy drinks, and sweetened teas contain added sugars that can contribute to weight gain, insulin resistance, and increased risk of heart disease.

• Processed Foods: Many processed foods like cereals, snacks, desserts, and sweetened condiments contain high amounts of added sugars, which should be limited.

4. High Sodium Foods:

• Processed and Packaged Foods: Fast food, frozen meals, canned soups, processed snacks, and condiments often have high sodium content, which can increase blood pressure and the risk of heart disease.

5. Refined Carbohydrates:

• White Bread, White Rice, and Pastries: Refined grains lack fiber and essential nutrients found in whole grains and may contribute to increased risk of heart disease and weight gain.

6. Excessive Alcohol:

• Heavy Drinking: Consuming excessive amounts of alcohol can raise blood pressure, increase triglycerides, and contribute to heart failure and other heart-related complications.

7. Excessive Salt:

• High-Sodium Condiments: Soy sauce, ketchup, and other high-sodium condiments can significantly increase daily salt intake, contributing to hypertension and heart disease.

8. Processed Snacks and Fast Foods:

• Chips, French Fries, and Snack Foods: These often contain unhealthy fats, high sodium, and trans fats that negatively impact heart health.

Moderation and portion control are crucial even with foods that might not be entirely avoided. While it's essential to limit or avoid these foods for better heart health, focusing on a well-rounded, balanced diet consisting of whole foods, fruits, vegetables, lean proteins, whole grains, and healthy fats is key to supporting cardiovascular wellness.

# HOW TO TAILOR THE MIND DIET FOR DIFFERENT DIETARY PREFERENCES

Adapting the MIND diet to different dietary preferences involves making adjustments while maintaining the core principles of the diet, which emphasize brain health and potentially support heart health. Here's how you can tailor the MIND diet for various dietary preferences:

1. Vegetarian or Vegan Preferences:

• Focus on Plant-Based Foods: Emphasize a variety of fruits, vegetables, legumes, nuts, seeds, and whole grains.

• Plant Protein Sources: Incorporate tofu, tempeh, lentils, chickpeas, beans, and edamame for protein.

• Omega-3 Sources: Include plant-based sources of omega-3 fatty acids like chia seeds, flaxseeds, walnuts, and algae-based supplements.

• Avoidance of Animal Products: Omit or limit animal products such as meat, poultry, fish, dairy, and eggs based on your specific dietary preference.

2. Gluten-Free Preferences:

• Choose Gluten-Free Whole Grains: Opt for gluten-free whole grains like quinoa, brown rice, amaranth, buckwheat, and certified gluten-free oats.

• Avoid Gluten-Containing Foods: Eliminate foods containing wheat, barley, rye, and other gluten-containing grains.

3. Low-Carb or Keto Preferences:

• Focus on Low-Carb Vegetables: Include non-starchy vegetables like leafy greens, broccoli, cauliflower, zucchini, and peppers.

• Healthy Fats: Incorporate avocados, olive oil, nuts, seeds, and fatty fish for healthy fats.

• Limit Carbohydrates: Reduce or eliminate high-carb foods like grains, legumes, fruits, and starchy vegetables according to your desired carb intake.

4. Paleo Preferences:

• Emphasize Whole Foods: Include lean meats, fish, seafood, eggs, nuts, seeds, fruits, and non-starchy vegetables.

• Avoid Processed Foods: Eliminate processed foods, refined sugars, grains, and legumes commonly restricted in the paleo diet.

5. Allergies or Sensitivities:

• Substitute Allergens: Replace allergenic foods with suitable alternatives. For example, if allergic to nuts, use seeds or other non-allergenic sources of healthy fats.

• Read Labels Carefully: Ensure foods and ingredients do not contain allergens you need to avoid.

6. Intermittent Fasting Preferences:

• Adjust Meal Timing: Structure eating windows according to your fasting schedule while incorporating MIND diet principles during eating periods.

• Focus on Nutrient Density: Consume nutrient-dense foods during eating windows to support brain and heart health.

7. Customization for Personal Taste:

• Flexibility in Food Choices: Modify specific food selections within the MIND diet framework to suit personal preferences while ensuring nutritional adequacy.

• Experiment with Recipes: Adapt MIND diet recipes to incorporate preferred flavors or ingredients while maintaining the overall nutrient profile.

Consulting a registered dietitian or healthcare professional can provide personalized guidance based on individual dietary preferences and health goals while adhering to the principles of the MIND diet to promote brain health and potentially support heart health.

## HOW TO TAILOR THE MIND DIET FOR DIFFERENT CULTURAL BACKGROUNDS

Adapting the MIND diet to different cultural backgrounds involves incorporating the core principles of the diet while allowing for flexibility in food choices to align with diverse cultural cuisines and preferences. Here's how you can tailor the MIND diet for various cultural backgrounds:

1. Embrace Diversity in Plant-Based Foods:

• Include Culturally Relevant Fruits and Vegetables: Incorporate a wide variety of fruits and vegetables commonly found in your cultural cuisine. For instance, Mediterranean diets might include olives, figs, and artichokes, while Asian cuisines often feature bok choy, daikon, and lychees.

• Explore Local Produce: Use locally available produce to integrate traditional flavors into MIND diet recipes.

2. Adapt Protein Sources:

• Select Traditional Protein Sources: Choose lean meats, fish, poultry, or plant-based proteins according to cultural preferences. For example, Mediterranean diets often include fish and legumes, while Asian diets may include tofu, tempeh, or lean cuts of meat.

• Incorporate Cultural Spices and Herbs: Use traditional spices and herbs to flavor proteins, enhancing taste while aligning with cultural preferences.

3. Incorporate Whole Grains:

• Explore Indigenous Whole Grains: Integrate traditional whole grains or pseudo-cereals such as quinoa, amaranth, millet, or teff that align with cultural backgrounds into meals.

• Replace with Local Alternatives: Substitute familiar grains in the MIND diet recipes with culturally relevant whole grains or their equivalents.

4. Utilize Healthy Fats:

• Cultural Cooking Oils: Use traditional cooking oils (e.g., olive oil in Mediterranean cuisine, sesame oil in Asian cuisine) to incorporate healthy fats into meals.

5. Accommodate Dietary Restrictions:

• Adapt Recipes for Allergies or Sensitivities: Modify MIND diet recipes to accommodate specific dietary restrictions, using alternative ingredients while respecting cultural traditions.

• Customize Based on Dietary Needs: Tailor the MIND diet to include foods that meet dietary needs while aligning with cultural values and customs.

6. Preserve Culinary Practices:

• Maintain Cooking Techniques: Retain traditional cooking methods and techniques that are characteristic of cultural cuisines while preparing MIND diet-friendly meals.

• Promote Culinary Traditions: Embrace and celebrate cultural food traditions by integrating them into a MIND diet framework.

7. Foster Community and Sharing:

• Social Aspects of Eating: Emphasize the social and communal aspects of mealtime, which are often central to many cultural dining experiences.

• Celebrate Food Diversity: Embrace and share diverse cultural foods and recipes with friends and family, incorporating MIND diet principles.

Ultimately, tailoring the MIND diet to different cultural backgrounds involves a thoughtful integration of traditional foods, cooking methods, and dietary practices while promoting the fundamental principles of the diet to support brain health and potentially enhance heart health. Consulting with a registered dietitian familiar with both cultural diversity and nutritional science can provide personalized guidance for adapting the MIND diet to specific cultural preferences and dietary needs.

## HOW TO TAILOR THE MIND DIET FOR DIFFERENT LIFESTYLES

Adapting the MIND diet to different lifestyles involves incorporating its core principles while making adjustments to accommodate varying schedules, preferences, and eating habits. Here's how you can tailor the MIND diet for different lifestyles:

1. Busy or On-the-Go Lifestyles:

• Meal Prep and Planning: Schedule time for meal planning and preparation to ensure access to MIND diet-friendly foods during busy days.

• Convenient Healthy Snacks: Pack portable snacks like nuts, seeds, fresh fruits, or pre-cut veggies to maintain healthy eating habits while on the go.

• Quick and Easy Recipes: Opt for simple and quick MIND diet recipes that require minimal cooking time but still incorporate nutritious ingredients.

2. Active Lifestyles:

• Nutrient-Dense Foods: Prioritize foods rich in antioxidants, healthy fats, and proteins to support energy levels and recovery for active individuals.

• Balanced Meals: Incorporate a combination of lean proteins, whole grains, and colorful fruits and vegetables to fuel workouts and aid in muscle recovery.

3. Vegetarian or Vegan Lifestyles:

• Plant-Based Protein Sources: Explore diverse plant-based protein options like beans, lentils, tofu, tempeh, and quinoa to ensure adequate protein intake.

• Omega-3 Sources: Include flaxseeds, chia seeds, walnuts, and algae-based supplements for plant-based omega-3 fatty acids.

4. Intermittent Fasting:

• Timing of Meals: Adjust meal timing during eating windows to align with intermittent fasting schedules while ensuring nutrient-dense MIND diet meals.

5. Seniors or Older Adults:

• Nutrient-Dense Foods: Prioritize easy-to-chew and nutrient-rich foods like smoothies, soups, and soft-cooked vegetables for easier digestion.

• Portion Control: Adjust portion sizes to meet individual energy needs while ensuring a balanced intake of nutrients recommended by the MIND diet.

6. Weight Management Goals:

• Portion Control and Caloric Awareness: Monitor portion sizes and caloric intake while focusing on nutrient-dense foods to support weight management within the MIND diet framework.

• Balanced Approach: Emphasize whole foods and mindful eating practices to maintain a healthy weight while following the principles of the MIND diet.

7. Social Lifestyles:

• Flexible Dining Choices: Adapt MIND diet principles when dining out by choosing restaurants with healthier options or making informed choices while enjoying social meals.

• Sharing Healthy Recipes: Incorporate MIND diet-friendly recipes when hosting social gatherings or potlucks to promote healthy eating among friends and family.

8. Customization for Personal Preferences:

• Flexibility in Food Choices: Modify specific food selections within the MIND diet framework to suit personal preferences while ensuring nutritional adequacy.

• Experiment with Recipes: Adapt MIND diet recipes to incorporate preferred flavors or ingredients while maintaining the overall nutrient profile.

Tailoring the MIND diet for different lifestyles involves finding a balance between the diet's core principles and individual preferences, schedules, and nutritional needs. Consulting with a registered dietitian or healthcare professional can provide personalized guidance tailored to specific lifestyles while aligning with the principles of the MIND diet for optimal brain and potential heart health.

## PRACTICAL TIPS AND STRATEGIES TO HELP INDIVIDUALS ADHERE TO THE MIND DIET FOR HEART HEALTH

Adherence to the MIND diet for heart health can be facilitated by implementing practical strategies and incorporating small changes into daily routines. Here are some practical tips to help individuals adhere to the MIND diet:

1. Gradual Changes:

• Start Small: Begin by gradually incorporating MIND diet principles into meals rather than attempting drastic changes all at once.

• Make Substitutions: Replace unhealthy options with MIND diet-approved alternatives, such as swapping refined grains for whole grains or unhealthy fats for healthier options like olive oil.

2. Meal Planning and Preparation:

• Plan Ahead: Schedule meal planning and preparation time to ensure MIND diet-friendly foods are readily available.

• Batch Cooking: Prepare larger portions and batch-cook MIND diet meals for the week to save time and ensure healthier eating choices.

3. Emphasize Fruits and Vegetables:

• Variety is Key: Aim for diverse colors and types of fruits and vegetables daily to maximize nutrient intake.

• Convenience Matters: Keep pre-cut vegetables or pre-washed fruits easily accessible for quick and healthy snacking options.

4. Healthy Snacking:

• Smart Snacking: Opt for nuts, seeds, yogurt, or fresh fruits as healthy snack choices, avoiding processed and high-sugar snacks.

• Portion Control: Be mindful of portion sizes, even with healthy snacks, to maintain balance.

5. Whole Grains and Legumes:

• Swap Refined Grains: Replace white bread, rice, and pasta with whole grain alternatives like brown rice, quinoa, or whole wheat options.

• Include Legumes: Incorporate beans, lentils, and chickpeas into soups, salads, or main dishes for added fiber and nutrients.

6. Healthy Fats:

• Use Healthy Oils: Cook with olive oil or avocado oil instead of saturated or trans fats.

• Add Nuts and Seeds: Include almonds, walnuts, flaxseeds, or chia seeds in meals or snacks for healthy fats.

7. Seafood Consumption:

• Increase Omega-3 Intake: Aim for at least two servings of fatty fish per week to meet omega-3 fatty acid recommendations.

• Diversify Seafood Choices: Incorporate different types of fish like salmon, mackerel, sardines, or trout for variety.

8. Limit Processed and Unhealthy Foods:

• Read Labels: Be mindful of added sugars, unhealthy fats, and sodium content in processed foods, and try to minimize their consumption.

• Smart Eating Out: When dining out, choose restaurants with healthier options or make informed choices to align with the MIND diet principles.

9. Stay Hydrated:

• Water Intake: Ensure adequate hydration throughout the day by drinking water and minimizing sugary beverages.

10. Mindful Eating:

• Savor Meals: Eat slowly, enjoy the flavors, and pay attention to hunger and fullness cues to prevent overeating.

• Practice Moderation: Indulge in less healthy foods occasionally but in moderation, without compromising overall adherence to the MIND diet.

11. Support and Accountability:

• Seek Support: Join support groups or involve family and friends in adopting healthier eating habits to stay motivated and accountable.

• Track Progress: Use food journals or apps to track meals, making it easier to monitor adherence and identify areas for improvement.

Incorporating these practical strategies into daily routines can help individuals gradually adopt and maintain the MIND diet for heart health, making it a sustainable lifestyle change for overall well-being. Consulting a registered dietitian or healthcare professional can offer personalized guidance and support in implementing the MIND diet effectively.

## THE IMPORTANCE OF REGULAR PHYSICAL ACTIVITY IN CONJUNCTION WITH A HEALTHY DIET FOR OPTIMAL HEART HEALTH

Regular physical activity plays a crucial role in maintaining optimal heart health when combined with a healthy diet like the MIND diet. Here's why it's essential and how it complements a nutritious eating plan:

1. Cardiovascular Health:

• Improves Heart Function: Regular exercise strengthens the heart muscle, enhances blood circulation, and improves cardiovascular endurance.

• Lowers Risk of Heart Disease: Physical activity helps lower blood pressure, reduce LDL ("bad") cholesterol, increase HDL ("good") cholesterol, and manage weight—all factors linked to a lower risk of heart disease.

2. Weight Management:

• Aids in Weight Control: Combining a healthy diet with regular physical activity supports weight loss or maintenance, reducing the risk of obesity-related heart issues.

3. Blood Sugar Regulation:

• Enhances Insulin Sensitivity: Exercise helps regulate blood sugar levels, reducing the risk of insulin resistance and type 2 diabetes, which are linked to heart disease.

4. Overall Health Benefits:

• Reduces Inflammation: Physical activity helps reduce systemic inflammation, which is associated with various chronic diseases, including heart disease.

• Boosts Mood and Reduces Stress: Regular exercise releases endorphins, improving mood, reducing stress, and indirectly benefiting heart health.

5. Synergy with a Healthy Diet:

• Enhances Diet Benefits: Pairing a healthy diet like the MIND diet with regular physical activity amplifies the overall heart-protective effects, promoting optimal health outcomes.

• Balanced Lifestyle: Combining nutritious eating habits with exercise creates a well-rounded approach to heart health, supporting a balanced and healthy lifestyle.

Recommendations for Physical Activity:

• Aerobic Exercise: Engage in moderate-intensity aerobic activities like brisk walking, cycling, swimming, or dancing for at least 150 minutes per week or aim for 75 minutes of vigorous-intensity aerobic activity per week.

• Strength Training: Incorporate strength or resistance training exercises for major muscle groups at least twice a week.

• Flexibility and Balance: Include flexibility and balance exercises to improve overall fitness and reduce the risk of injury, enhancing overall physical well-being.

Importance of Consistency:

• Long-Term Benefits: Consistency in physical activity is key to reaping long-term heart health benefits. Regular exercise becomes a lifestyle habit that supports heart health and overall well-being.

In conclusion, regular physical activity is a fundamental component of maintaining optimal heart health. When combined with a healthy diet like the MIND diet, exercise enhances cardiovascular fitness, aids in weight management, regulates blood sugar levels, reduces inflammation, and contributes to overall well-being, forming a comprehensive approach to heart health and disease prevention.

# THE IMPACT OF STRESS MANAGEMENT TECHNIqUES AND SUFFICIENT SLEEP ON HEART HEALTH IN RELATION TO DIET

Stress management techniques and sufficient sleep are integral components of heart health, and when combined with a healthy diet like the MIND diet, they play essential roles in reducing the risk of heart disease. Here's their impact and how they relate to diet:

Stress Management:

• Effect on Eating Habits: Chronic stress can lead to unhealthy eating patterns, including overeating or choosing high-fat and high-sugar comfort foods, which may negatively impact heart health.

• Influence on Heart Health: Prolonged stress increases the risk of high blood pressure, inflammation, and heart disease, making stress management crucial for heart health.

• Relation to Diet: Stress-reducing techniques like meditation, deep breathing exercises, yoga, or mindfulness practices can positively impact eating behaviors and adherence to a healthy diet, including the MIND diet.

Sufficient Sleep:

• Sleep Quality and Heart Health: Inadequate sleep or poor sleep quality is associated with an increased risk of hypertension, weight gain, insulin resistance, and heart disease.

• Impact on Dietary Choices: Lack of sleep can disrupt hormones regulating appetite and cravings, leading to increased consumption of unhealthy foods and reduced adherence to a healthy diet.

• Connection to Diet: A well-rested body is better equipped to regulate hunger hormones, make healthier food choices, and maintain consistent energy levels to support adherence to a heart-healthy diet like the MIND diet.

Strategies for Stress Management and Better Sleep:

• Mindfulness Practices: Incorporate mindfulness meditation, deep breathing exercises, or yoga into daily routines to reduce stress levels.

• Establish Sleep Routine: Maintain a regular sleep schedule, create a relaxing bedtime routine, and ensure a conducive sleep environment for better sleep quality.

Synergy with a Healthy Diet:

• Complementary Effects: Stress management and adequate sleep complement a healthy diet by promoting overall well-being, reducing the risk factors associated with heart disease, and enhancing the positive effects of a nutritious eating plan like the MIND diet.

• Holistic Approach: Adopting stress-reduction techniques and prioritizing sufficient sleep alongside a healthy diet creates a holistic approach to heart health, addressing multiple factors that contribute to cardiovascular wellness.

Lifestyle Balance for Heart Health:

• Balance and Harmony: A balanced approach that integrates stress management, sufficient sleep, and a healthy diet fosters an environment conducive to heart health.

• Supporting Each Other: Stress management and better sleep support adherence to a healthy diet by creating a more conducive environment for making mindful food choices and sustaining healthy eating habits.

In summary, stress management techniques and sufficient sleep are critical components of heart health. They work synergistically with a healthy diet, such as the MIND diet, by influencing eating behaviors, reducing risk factors for heart disease, and supporting overall well-being, fostering a holistic approach to maintaining cardiovascular wellness.

# CHAPTER TWO



Berry and Yogurt Parfait

Ingredients:

- 1 cup Greek yogurt (unsweetened)

- ½ cup mixed berries (blueberries, strawberries, raspberries)

- ¼ cup granola (preferably low-sugar or homemade)

- 1 tablespoon honey or maple syrup (optional)

Instructions:

1. In a glass or bowl, layer the Greek yogurt at the bottom.

2. Add a layer of mixed berries on top of the yogurt. Sprinkle granola over the berries.

3. Repeat layers as desired. Drizzle honey or maple syrup for added sweetness if desired.

4. Serve immediately.

# Veggie Omelette

Ingredients:

- 2 eggs

- 1 tablespoon olive oil

- ½ cup chopped mixed vegetables (spinach, bell peppers, tomatoes, mushrooms)

- Salt and pepper to taste

- 2 tablespoons grated low-fat cheese (optional)

Instructions:

1. In a bowl, whisk eggs until well beaten. Season with salt and pepper.

2. Heat olive oil in a non-stick skillet over medium heat. Add chopped vegetables to the skillet and sauté until tender.

3. Pour beaten eggs over the vegetables and cook until the edges start to set.

4. Gently lift the edges of the omelette and let the uncooked eggs flow underneath to cook evenly. Sprinkle grated cheese over the omelette if using.

5. Fold the omelette in half and cook for another minute until the cheese melts. Slide onto a plate and serve hot.

Overnight Chia Seed Pudding

Ingredients:

• 2 tablespoons chia seeds

• ½ cup unsweetened almond milk (or any milk of choice)

• ¼ teaspoon vanilla extract

• ½ tablespoon honey or maple syrup (optional)

• Sliced fruits and nuts for topping

Instructions:

1. In a jar or bowl, mix chia seeds, almond milk, vanilla extract, and sweetener (if using). Stir well.

2. Cover the jar or bowl and refrigerate overnight or for at least 4 hours until it thickens.

3. Before serving, stir the chia seed mixture. Add more milk if desired for a thinner consistency.

4. Top with sliced fruits and nuts before serving.

Whole Grain Toast with Avocado and Tomato

Ingredients:

• 2 slices whole grain bread (toasted)

• 1 ripe avocado (mashed)

• 1 tomato (sliced)

• Salt and pepper to taste

• Optional: A sprinkle of red pepper flakes or fresh herbs

Instructions:

1. Toast the whole grain bread slices until golden brown. Spread mashed avocado evenly on each slice.

2. Arrange sliced tomatoes on top of the avocado. Season with salt, pepper, and any additional desired toppings.

3. Serve immediately.


Greek Yogurt and Fruit Smoothie

Ingredients:

• 1 cup Greek yogurt (unsweetened)

• 1 ripe banana (frozen)

- ½ cup mixed berries (frozen or fresh)

- ½ cup spinach or kale leaves (optional)

- 1 tablespoon honey or maple syrup (optional)

- ½ cup water or unsweetened almond milk

Instructions:

1. In a blender, combine Greek yogurt, frozen banana, mixed berries, optional greens, sweetener (if using), and liquid (water or almond milk).

2. Blend until smooth and creamy.

3. Pour into a glass and serve immediately.

## Spinach and Feta Egg Muffins

Ingredients:

- 6 eggs

- 1 cup fresh spinach (chopped)

- 1/4 cup feta cheese (crumbled)

- 1/4 cup red bell pepper (diced)

- Salt and pepper to taste

Instructions:

1. Preheat oven to 350°F (175°C) and grease a muffin tin.

2. In a mixing bowl, beat the eggs and season with salt and pepper.

3. Stir in chopped spinach, feta cheese, and diced red bell pepper into the egg mixture.

4. Pour the mixture evenly into the muffin tin. Bake for 20-25 minutes or until the egg muffins are set and slightly golden.

5. Allow them to cool slightly before removing from the muffin tin. Serve warm.


Apple Cinnamon Quinoa Porridge

Ingredients:

- 1/2 cup quinoa (rinsed)

- 1 cup unsweetened almond milk (or any milk of choice)

- 1 apple (diced)

- 1/2 teaspoon cinnamon

- 1 tablespoon honey or maple syrup (optional)

- Sliced almonds or walnuts for topping

Instructions:

1. In a saucepan, combine quinoa and almond milk. Bring to a boil, then reduce heat to low and simmer for 15-20 minutes until quinoa is cooked and liquid is absorbed.

2. Stir in diced apples, cinnamon, and sweetener (if using). Cook for an additional 5 minutes until apples are tender.

3. Remove from heat and let it sit for a few minutes. Adjust sweetness if needed.

4. Serve the quinoa porridge topped with sliced almonds or walnuts.

Avocado and Egg Breakfast Wrap

Ingredients:

• 1 whole grain tortilla or wrap

• 1 ripe avocado (sliced or mashed)

• 1 boiled egg (sliced)

• Handful of spinach leaves

• Sliced tomato

• Salt and pepper to taste

Instructions:

1. Lay the tortilla flat and spread mashed or sliced avocado over the surface.

2. Layer spinach leaves, sliced boiled egg, and tomato slices on top of the avocado. Season with salt and pepper.

3. Roll up the tortilla to create a wrap.

4. Optionally, grill or warm the wrap in a skillet for a few minutes. Slice in half and serve.


Blueberry Oatmeal Breakfast Bars

Ingredients:

• 2 cups rolled oats

• 1 cup mashed bananas (about 2-3 ripe bananas)

• 1/2 cup unsweetened applesauce

• 1/4 cup honey or maple syrup

• 1 teaspoon vanilla extract

• 1/2 teaspoon cinnamon

• 1 cup fresh or frozen blueberries

Instructions:

1. Preheat oven to 350°F (175°C) and line a baking pan with parchment paper.

2. In a mixing bowl, combine oats, mashed bananas, applesauce, honey or maple syrup, vanilla extract, and cinnamon. Mix until well combined.

3. Gently fold in blueberries.

4. Spread the mixture evenly into the prepared baking pan. Bake for 25-30 minutes or until the bars are set and golden brown.

5. Allow to cool completely before cutting into bars. Serve as a grab-and-go breakfast option.

## Mediterranean Breakfast Bowl

Ingredients:

• 1 cup cooked quinoa or bulgur wheat

• 1/4 cup cherry tomatoes (halved)

• 2 tablespoons diced cucumber

• 2 tablespoons chopped Kalamata olives

• 2 tablespoons crumbled feta cheese

- 1 tablespoon chopped fresh parsley

- 1 tablespoon extra virgin olive oil

- 1 teaspoon lemon juice

- Salt and pepper to taste

Instructions:

1. In a bowl, combine cooked quinoa or bulgur wheat with cherry tomatoes, diced cucumber, Kalamata olives, crumbled feta cheese, and fresh parsley.

2. Drizzle with extra virgin olive oil and lemon juice.

3. Season with salt and pepper to taste. Toss gently to combine all ingredients.

4. Serve the Mediterranean breakfast bowl fresh.


Sweet Potato Breakfast Hash

Ingredients:

- 1 large sweet potato (diced)

- 1 bell pepper (diced)

- 1 small onion (chopped)

- 2 cloves garlic (minced)

- 2 tablespoons olive oil

- 1 teaspoon smoked paprika

- Salt and pepper to taste

- 2 eggs (optional)

Instructions:

1. Heat olive oil in a skillet over medium heat. Add diced sweet potato and cook for 5-7 minutes until slightly softened.

2. Add diced bell pepper, chopped onion, and minced garlic to the skillet. Cook for an additional 5-7 minutes until vegetables are tender.

3. Sprinkle smoked paprika, salt, and pepper over the hash. Stir to combine and cook for another 2-3 minutes.

4. If desired, create wells in the hash and crack eggs into the wells. Cover and cook for 5-7 minutes until the eggs are set (optional).

5. Serve the sweet potato breakfast hash hot.

Veggie Breakfast Burrito

Ingredients:

• 2 whole grain tortillas or wraps

• 2 eggs (scrambled)

• 1/2 cup black beans (cooked)

• 1/4 cup diced tomatoes

• 1/4 cup diced bell peppers

• 2 tablespoons chopped cilantro

• 2 tablespoons shredded low-fat cheese

• Salsa or avocado (optional, for serving)

Instructions:

1. Lay tortillas flat and divide scrambled eggs between the two.

2. Top each tortilla with black beans, diced tomatoes, diced bell peppers, cilantro, and shredded cheese.

3. Optionally, add salsa or avocado slices for added flavor.

4. Roll up the tortillas to form burritos. Optionally, warm the burritos in a skillet for a few minutes.

5. Slice in half and serve.

Salmon and Avocado Toast

Ingredients:

- 2 slices whole grain bread (toasted)

- 1/2 avocado (sliced or mashed)

- 3-4 ounces smoked salmon

- Squeeze of lemon juice

- Fresh dill or parsley (for garnish)

- Salt and pepper to taste

Instructions:

1. Toast the whole grain bread slices until golden brown.

2. Spread sliced or mashed avocado evenly on each slice. Top with smoked salmon slices.

3. Squeeze fresh lemon juice over the salmon. Season with salt and pepper.

4. Garnish with fresh dill or parsley. Serve the salmon and avocado toast immediately.

Banana Walnut Breakfast Cookies

Ingredients:

• 2 ripe bananas (mashed)

• 1 cup rolled oats

• 1/4 cup chopped walnuts

• 2 tablespoons honey or maple syrup

• 1/2 teaspoon cinnamon

• 1/4 teaspoon vanilla extract

• Pinch of salt

Instructions:

1. Preheat oven to 350°F (175°C) and line a baking sheet with parchment paper.

2. In a bowl, mix mashed bananas, rolled oats, chopped walnuts, honey or maple syrup, cinnamon, vanilla extract, and a pinch of salt until well combined.

3. Scoop spoonfuls of the mixture and place them on the baking sheet, flattening them slightly to form cookies.

4. Bake for 15-18 minutes until golden brown and set.

5. Allow the banana walnut breakfast cookies to cool before serving.


Quinoa Breakfast Bowl with Berries

Ingredients:

• 1 cup cooked quinoa

• 1/2 cup mixed berries (strawberries, blueberries, raspberries)

• 2 tablespoons Greek yogurt

• 1 tablespoon honey or maple syrup

• 1 tablespoon chopped nuts (almonds, walnuts)

• Optional: Dash of cinnamon

Instructions:

1. In a bowl, layer cooked quinoa as the base.

2. Top with mixed berries and Greek yogurt.

3. Drizzle honey or maple syrup over the berries and yogurt. Sprinkle chopped nuts and a dash of cinnamon if desired.

4. Serve the quinoa breakfast bowl fresh.

Berry Spinach Smoothie Bowl

Ingredients:

• 1 cup spinach leaves

• 1 frozen banana

• 1/2 cup mixed berries (strawberries, blueberries, raspberries)

• 1/2 cup unsweetened almond milk (or any milk of choice)

• 2 tablespoons Greek yogurt

• Toppings: Sliced fruits, nuts, seeds, granola

Instructions:

1. In a blender, combine spinach, frozen banana, mixed berries, almond milk, and Greek yogurt.

2. Blend until smooth and creamy.

3. Pour the smoothie into a bowl. Top with sliced fruits, nuts, seeds, or granola for added texture and nutrients.

4. Enjoy the berry spinach smoothie bowl with a spoon.

Quinoa Breakfast Casserole

Ingredients:

• 1 cup cooked quinoa

• 1 cup diced vegetables (bell peppers, spinach, onions)

• 4 eggs

• 1/2 cup unsweetened almond milk (or any milk of choice)

• 1/2 cup shredded low-fat cheese

• Salt, pepper, and herbs of choice

Instructions:

1. Preheat oven to 350°F (175°C) and grease a baking dish.

2. Spread cooked quinoa evenly in the baking dish. Scatter diced vegetables over the quinoa.

3. In a separate bowl, whisk together eggs, almond milk, salt, pepper, and herbs.

4. Pour the egg mixture over the quinoa and vegetables in the baking dish. Sprinkle shredded cheese over the top.

5. Bake for 25-30 minutes until the casserole is set and the cheese is melted.

6. Allow it to cool slightly before slicing and serving.

Almond Butter and Banana Toast

Ingredients:

- 2 slices whole grain bread (toasted)

- 2 tablespoons almond butter

- 1 ripe banana (sliced)

- Optional: Drizzle of honey or sprinkle of cinnamon

Instructions:

1. Toast the whole grain bread slices until golden brown.

2. Spread almond butter evenly on each slice.

3. Arrange banana slices on top of the almond butter. Optionally, drizzle honey or sprinkle cinnamon for added sweetness and flavor.

4. Serve the almond butter and banana toast immediately.

Egg and Veggie Breakfast Quesadilla

Ingredients:

• 2 whole grain tortillas

• 2 eggs (scrambled)

• 1/2 cup diced vegetables (bell peppers, tomatoes, onions)

• 1/4 cup shredded low-fat cheese

• Optional: Salsa or Greek yogurt (for serving)

Instructions:

1. Heat a non-stick skillet over medium heat.

2. Place one tortilla in the skillet. Spread scrambled eggs, diced vegetables, and shredded cheese over the tortilla.

3. Place the second tortilla on top. Cook for 2-3 minutes on each side until the tortilla is golden and the cheese is melted.

4. Remove from heat, let it cool slightly, and slice into wedges.

5. Serve the egg and veggie breakfast quesadilla with salsa or Greek yogurt if desired.

Overnight Oats with Apples and Cinnamon

Ingredients:

• 1/2 cup rolled oats

• 1/2 cup unsweetened almond milk (or any milk of choice)

• 1/2 cup Greek yogurt

• 1 apple (diced)

• 1 tablespoon honey or maple syrup

• 1/2 teaspoon cinnamon

• Optional toppings: Sliced almonds, raisins, chia seeds

Instructions:

1. In a jar or bowl, combine rolled oats, almond milk, Greek yogurt, diced apple, honey or maple syrup, and cinnamon. Stir well.

2. Cover and refrigerate the mixture overnight or for at least 4 hours.

3. Before serving, stir the oats mixture and add more almond milk if desired for a thinner consistency.

4. Top with sliced almonds, raisins, or chia seeds for added texture and nutrients.

5. Enjoy the apple cinnamon overnight oats cold or at room temperature.


Green Shakshuka

Ingredients:

• 2 cups spinach leaves

• 1 cup kale leaves

• 1 tablespoon olive oil

• 2 cloves garlic (minced)

• 1/2 onion (chopped)

• 1 bell pepper (diced)

• 4 eggs

• Salt and pepper to taste

• Optional: Feta cheese, chopped herbs (parsley, cilantro)

Instructions:

1. Heat olive oil in a skillet over medium heat. Add minced garlic and chopped onion, sauté until fragrant.

2. Add diced bell pepper, spinach, and kale to the skillet. Cook until wilted.

3. Create small wells in the greens and crack eggs into each well. Cover and cook for 5-7 minutes until the eggs are set to desired doneness.

4. Season with salt and pepper. Optionally, sprinkle crumbled feta cheese and chopped herbs on top.

5. Serve the green shakshuka hot.


Coconut Chia Seed Pudding

Ingredients:

• 1/4 cup chia seeds

• 1 cup unsweetened coconut milk

• 1 tablespoon honey or maple syrup

• 1/2 teaspoon vanilla extract

• Fresh fruits (such as berries, mango, or kiwi) for topping

• Unsweetened shredded coconut (optional)

Instructions:

1. In a bowl or jar, mix chia seeds, coconut milk, honey or maple syrup, and vanilla extract. Stir well.

2. Cover and refrigerate the mixture for at least 2 hours or overnight until it thickens.

3. Before serving, stir the chia seed pudding. Add more coconut milk if a thinner consistency is desired.

4. Top with fresh fruits and shredded coconut.

5. Enjoy the coconut chia seed pudding chilled.

Breakfast Quinoa with Berries

Ingredients:

• 1 cup cooked quinoa

• 1/2 cup mixed berries (blueberries, strawberries, raspberries)

• 2 tablespoons chopped nuts (almonds, walnuts)

• 1 tablespoon honey or maple syrup

• Dash of cinnamon

Instructions:

1. In a bowl, combine cooked quinoa and mixed berries.

2. Drizzle honey or maple syrup over the quinoa and berries. Sprinkle chopped nuts and a dash of cinnamon.

3. Mix all ingredients together.

4. Serve the breakfast quinoa with berries at room temperature or warmed.

Mediterranean Veggie Breakfast Skillet

Ingredients:

- 2 tablespoons olive oil

- 1/2 onion (chopped)

- 1 bell pepper (diced)

- 1 cup cherry tomatoes (halved)

- 2 cups spinach leaves

- 4 eggs

- Salt, pepper, and herbs (such as oregano or thyme) to taste

- Optional: Feta cheese, olives

Instructions:

1. Heat olive oil in a skillet over medium heat. Add chopped onion and bell pepper. Sauté until softened.

2. Add cherry tomatoes to the skillet and cook for a few minutes until they start to soften.

3. Stir in spinach leaves and cook until wilted.

4. Create wells in the vegetable mixture and crack eggs into each well. Cover and cook for 5-7 minutes until the eggs are cooked to desired doneness.

5. Season with salt, pepper, and herbs. Optionally, top with crumbled feta cheese and olives.

6. Serve the Mediterranean veggie breakfast skillet hot.


## Apple Cinnamon Baked Oatmeal Cups

Ingredients:

• 2 cups rolled oats

• 1 teaspoon baking powder

• 1 teaspoon cinnamon

• 1/4 teaspoon salt

- 1 1/2 cups unsweetened almond milk

- 2 tablespoons honey or maple syrup

- 1 large apple (diced)

- Chopped nuts for topping (optional)

Instructions:

1. Preheat oven to 350°F (175°C) and grease a muffin tin.

2. In a bowl, mix rolled oats, baking powder, cinnamon, and salt.

3. Add almond milk, honey or maple syrup, and diced apple to the dry ingredients. Mix well.

4. Spoon the mixture into the muffin tin, filling each cup. Sprinkle chopped nuts on top if using.

5. Bake for 25-30 minutes until the oatmeal cups are set and golden.

6. Allow them to cool slightly before removing from the muffin tin.

7. Serve the apple cinnamon baked oatmeal cups warm or at room temperature.

Mediterranean Chickpea Salad

Ingredients:

• 1 can (15 oz) chickpeas (drained and rinsed)

• 1 cucumber (diced)

• 1 cup cherry tomatoes (halved)

• 1/4 cup red onion (finely chopped)

• 1/4 cup Kalamata olives (pitted and halved)

• 2 tablespoons chopped fresh parsley

• 2 tablespoons extra virgin olive oil

• 1 tablespoon lemon juice

• Salt and pepper to taste

• Optional: Feta cheese

Instructions:

1. In a large bowl, combine chickpeas, diced cucumber, cherry tomatoes, red onion, Kalamata olives, and chopped parsley.

2. Drizzle extra virgin olive oil and lemon juice over the salad. Season with salt and pepper, then toss gently to combine.

3. Optionally, sprinkle crumbled feta cheese on top.

4. Serve the Mediterranean chickpea salad chilled or at room temperature.

Grilled Lemon Herb Chicken Breast

Ingredients:

• 2 boneless, skinless chicken breasts

• 2 tablespoons olive oil

• 2 cloves garlic (minced)

• 1 teaspoon lemon zest

• 2 tablespoons fresh lemon juice

• 1 tablespoon chopped fresh herbs (rosemary, thyme, or oregano)

• Salt and pepper to taste

Instructions:

1. In a bowl, mix olive oil, minced garlic, lemon zest, lemon juice, fresh herbs, salt, and pepper.

2. Place chicken breasts in a shallow dish and pour the marinade over them, ensuring they're evenly coated. Marinate for at least 30 minutes.

3. Preheat grill or grill pan over medium-high heat.

4. Grill chicken breasts for about 6-7 minutes per side or until cooked through (internal temperature reaches 165°F or 74°C).

5. Remove from grill, let rest for a few minutes, then slice.

6. Serve the grilled lemon herb chicken breast with your choice of side salad or vegetables.

## Quinoa Stuffed Bell Peppers

Ingredients:

• 4 bell peppers (any color)

• 1 cup cooked quinoa

• 1 can (15 oz) black beans (drained and rinsed)

• 1 cup diced tomatoes

• 1/2 cup corn kernels (fresh, canned, or frozen)

• 1/4 cup chopped fresh cilantro

• 1 teaspoon ground cumin

- Salt and pepper to taste

- Optional: Shredded cheese

Instructions:

1. Preheat oven to 375°F (190°C). Slice the tops off the bell peppers and remove seeds and membranes.

2. In a bowl, mix cooked quinoa, black beans, diced tomatoes, corn kernels, chopped cilantro, ground cumin, salt, and pepper.

3. Stuff each bell pepper with the quinoa mixture.

4. Place the stuffed peppers in a baking dish. Optionally, sprinkle shredded cheese on top.

5. Cover the dish with foil and bake for 25-30 minutes until peppers are tender.

6. Remove foil and bake for an additional 5 minutes to melt the cheese (if using).

7. Serve the quinoa stuffed bell peppers hot.

Ingredients:

• 2 salmon fillets

• 2 cups mixed vegetables (such as broccoli, bell peppers, zucchini)

• 2 tablespoons olive oil

• 2 cloves garlic (minced)

• 1 tablespoon lemon juice

• Salt and pepper to taste

• Fresh herbs (parsley or dill) for garnish

Instructions:

1. Preheat oven to 400°F (200°C). Cut two large pieces of aluminum foil.

2. Place each salmon fillet on a piece of foil. Arrange mixed vegetables around the salmon.

3. In a small bowl, mix olive oil, minced garlic, lemon juice, salt, and pepper.

4. Drizzle the olive oil mixture evenly over the salmon and vegetables. Fold the foil over the salmon and veggies, crimping the edges to form sealed packets.

5. Place the foil packets on a baking sheet and bake for 15-20 minutes until salmon is cooked through and vegetables are tender.

6. Carefully open the packets, garnish with fresh herbs, and serve.

Veggie and Bean Burrito Bowl

Ingredients:

• 1 cup cooked brown rice or quinoa

• 1 can (15 oz) black beans (drained and rinsed)

• 1 cup diced tomatoes

• 1 avocado (sliced)

• 1/2 cup corn kernels (fresh, canned, or frozen)

• 1/4 cup chopped red onion

• 1/4 cup chopped cilantro

• Juice of 1 lime

• Salt and pepper to taste

• Optional: Salsa, Greek yogurt (as toppings)

Instructions:

1. In a bowl, mix cooked brown rice or quinoa, black beans, diced tomatoes, corn kernels, chopped red onion, chopped cilantro, lime juice, salt, and pepper.

2. Divide the mixture into serving bowls. Top each bowl with sliced avocado.

3. Optionally, add salsa or a dollop of Greek yogurt as toppings.

4. Serve the veggie and bean burrito bowls at room temperature.

## Lemon Garlic Shrimp with Quinoa

Ingredients:

• 1 pound shrimp (peeled and deveined)

• 2 tablespoons olive oil

• 3 cloves garlic (minced)

• Zest of 1 lemon

• Juice of 1 lemon

• 2 cups cooked quinoa

• 2 cups baby spinach leaves

• Salt and pepper to taste

• Fresh parsley for garnish

Instructions:

1. Heat olive oil in a skillet over medium heat. Add minced garlic and sauté for a minute.

2. Add shrimp to the skillet and cook until they turn pink, about 2-3 minutes per side.

3. Add lemon zest and lemon juice to the shrimp. Season with salt and pepper.

4. In a separate bowl, toss cooked quinoa with baby spinach until spinach begins to wilt.

5. Serve the lemon garlic shrimp over the quinoa and spinach mixture.

6. Garnish with fresh parsley and additional lemon wedges if desired.

## Turkey and Veggie Lettuce Wraps

Ingredients:

• 1 pound ground turkey

• 1 tablespoon olive oil

- 1/2 onion (chopped)

- 2 cloves garlic (minced)

- 1 bell pepper (diced)

- 1 cup shredded carrots

- 1/2 cup water chestnuts (chopped)

- 2 tablespoons low-sodium soy sauce

- 1 tablespoon hoisin sauce

- Lettuce leaves for wrapping (butter lettuce or iceberg lettuce)

Instructions:

1. Heat olive oil in a skillet over medium heat. Add chopped onion and minced garlic, sauté until fragrant.

2. Add ground turkey to the skillet and cook until browned.

3. Stir in diced bell pepper, shredded carrots, and chopped water chestnuts. Cook for a few minutes until vegetables soften.

4. Add low-sodium soy sauce and hoisin sauce, stir to combine.

5. Spoon the turkey and veggie mixture onto lettuce leaves, wrap them up, and secure with toothpicks if needed.

6. Serve the turkey and veggie lettuce wraps as a healthy lunch option.

## Tuna Salad Stuffed Avocado

Ingredients:

- 2 cans (5 oz each) tuna in water (drained)

- 2 ripe avocados

- 1/4 cup diced red onion

- 1/4 cup diced celery

- 1/4 cup diced cucumber

- 2 tablespoons Greek yogurt

- 1 tablespoon lemon juice

- Salt and pepper to taste

- Optional: Fresh herbs (such as parsley or dill)

Instructions:

1. In a bowl, mix drained tuna, diced red onion, diced celery, diced cucumber, Greek yogurt, lemon juice, salt, and pepper.

2. Cut ripe avocados in half and remove pits.

3. Scoop out some avocado flesh to create a larger hollow space for the tuna salad.

4. Fill each avocado half with the tuna salad mixture. Optionally, garnish with fresh herbs before serving.

Veggie Lentil Soup

Ingredients:

• 1 cup dried green or brown lentils (rinsed)

• 1 tablespoon olive oil

• 1 onion (chopped)

• 2 carrots (diced)

• 2 celery stalks (diced)

• 3 cloves garlic (minced)

• 6 cups vegetable broth

• 1 can (14 oz) diced tomatoes

• 1 teaspoon ground cumin

• 1 teaspoon paprika

• Salt and pepper to taste

- Fresh parsley for garnish

Instructions:

1. Heat olive oil in a large pot over medium heat. Add chopped onion, diced carrots, diced celery, and minced garlic. Sauté until vegetables soften.

2. Add rinsed lentils, vegetable broth, diced tomatoes (with juices), ground cumin, paprika, salt, and pepper to the pot.

3. Bring the mixture to a boil, then reduce heat to low. Simmer for about 25-30 minutes until lentils are tender.

4. Adjust seasoning if needed and garnish with fresh parsley before serving.

## Caprese Quinoa Salad

Ingredients:

- 2 cups cooked quinoa

- 1 cup cherry tomatoes (halved)

- 1 cup fresh mozzarella balls (mini size)

- 1/4 cup fresh basil leaves (chopped)

- 2 tablespoons extra virgin olive oil

- 1 tablespoon balsamic vinegar

- Salt and pepper to taste

Instructions:

1. In a large bowl, combine cooked quinoa, cherry tomatoes, fresh mozzarella balls, and chopped basil leaves.

2. Drizzle extra virgin olive oil and balsamic vinegar over the salad.

3. Season with salt and pepper, then toss gently to combine.

4. Serve the Caprese quinoa salad at room temperature or chilled.


Spinach and Chickpea Salad with Lemon Dressing

Ingredients:

- 2 cups fresh spinach leaves

- 1 can (15 oz) chickpeas (drained and rinsed)

- 1/4 cup sliced red onion

- 1/2 cup cherry tomatoes (halved)

- 1/4 cup crumbled feta cheese

• 2 tablespoons chopped fresh parsley

For the dressing:

• 2 tablespoons extra virgin olive oil

• Juice of 1 lemon

• 1 clove garlic (minced)

• Salt and pepper to taste

Instructions:

1. In a large bowl, combine fresh spinach leaves, chickpeas, sliced red onion, cherry tomatoes, crumbled feta cheese, and chopped fresh parsley.

2. In a separate small bowl, whisk together extra virgin olive oil, lemon juice, minced garlic, salt, and pepper to make the dressing.

3. Drizzle the dressing over the salad and toss gently to coat all ingredients.

4. Serve the spinach and chickpea salad immediately.

Ingredients:

• 4 bone-in, skinless chicken thighs

• 2 tablespoons olive oil

• Juice of 1 lemon

• Zest of 1 lemon

• 2 cloves garlic (minced)

• 1 teaspoon chopped fresh rosemary

• 1 teaspoon chopped fresh thyme

• Salt and pepper to taste

Instructions:

1. Preheat oven to 375°F (190°C) and line a baking dish with parchment paper.

2. In a bowl, mix together olive oil, lemon juice, lemon zest, minced garlic, chopped rosemary, chopped thyme, salt, and pepper.

3. Place chicken thighs in the prepared baking dish and pour the marinade over them, ensuring they are coated evenly.

4. Bake for 25-30 minutes until the chicken thighs are golden brown and cooked through (internal temperature reaches 165°F or 74°C).

5. Remove from the oven and let rest for a few minutes before serving.

Quinoa and Black Bean Stuffed Bell Peppers

Ingredients:

• 4 bell peppers (any color)

• 1 cup cooked quinoa

• 1 can (15 oz) black beans (drained and rinsed)

• 1 cup corn kernels (fresh, canned, or frozen)

• 1/2 cup diced tomatoes

• 1/4 cup chopped cilantro

• 1 teaspoon ground cumin

• Salt and pepper to taste

• Shredded cheese for topping (optional)

Instructions:

1. Preheat oven to 375°F (190°C). Cut the tops off the bell peppers and remove seeds.

2. In a bowl, mix together cooked quinoa, black beans, corn kernels, diced tomatoes, chopped cilantro, ground cumin, salt, and pepper.

3. Stuff each bell pepper with the quinoa and black bean mixture.

4. Place the stuffed peppers in a baking dish. Optionally, sprinkle shredded cheese on top.

5. Bake for 25-30 minutes until the peppers are tender.

6. Serve the quinoa and black bean stuffed bell peppers hot.

Grilled Vegetable Wrap with Hummus

Ingredients:

• Assorted vegetables (bell peppers, zucchini, eggplant, mushrooms)

• Whole grain wraps or tortillas

• 1/2 cup hummus

• Olive oil

• Salt and pepper to taste

Instructions:

1. Preheat grill or grill pan over medium-high heat. Slice vegetables into thin strips or rounds.

2. Brush vegetables with olive oil and season with salt and pepper.

3. Grill vegetables for a few minutes on each side until tender and lightly charred.

4. Warm wraps or tortillas on the grill for a minute. Spread hummus over each wrap, then place grilled vegetables on top.

5. Roll up the wraps and slice in half if desired.

6. Serve the grilled vegetable wrap with hummus immediately.

Lemon Garlic Shrimp Pasta

Ingredients:

• 8 oz whole grain spaghetti or pasta of choice

• 1 pound shrimp (peeled and deveined)

• 2 tablespoons olive oil

• 3 cloves garlic (minced)

- Zest of 1 lemon

- Juice of 1 lemon

- 1/4 cup chopped fresh parsley

- Salt and pepper to taste

- Optional: Grated Parmesan cheese

Instructions:

1. Cook pasta according to package instructions. Drain and set aside.

2. In a skillet, heat olive oil over medium heat. Add minced garlic and cook for a minute.

3. Add shrimp to the skillet and cook until they turn pink, about 2-3 minutes per side.

4. Add lemon zest, lemon juice, chopped fresh parsley, salt, and pepper to the shrimp. Toss to combine.

5. Add cooked pasta to the skillet with the shrimp and toss everything together.

6. Optionally, sprinkle grated Parmesan cheese on top before serving.

## Lentil and Vegetable Soup

Ingredients:

- 1 cup dried green or brown lentils (rinsed)

- 6 cups low-sodium vegetable broth

- 2 carrots (diced)

- 2 celery stalks (diced)

- 1 onion (chopped)

- 2 cloves garlic (minced)

- 1 can (14 oz) diced tomatoes

- 1 teaspoon ground cumin

- 1 teaspoon paprika

- Salt and pepper to taste

- Fresh parsley for garnish

Instructions:

1. In a large pot, combine rinsed lentils, vegetable broth, diced carrots, diced celery, chopped onion, minced garlic, diced tomatoes (with juices), ground cumin, paprika, salt, and pepper.

2. Bring the mixture to a boil, then reduce heat to low. Simmer for about 25-30 minutes until lentils are tender.

3. Adjust seasoning if needed and garnish with fresh parsley before serving.

Baked Salmon with Lemon and Herbs

Ingredients:

• 4 salmon fillets

• 2 tablespoons olive oil

• 2 cloves garlic (minced)

• Zest of 1 lemon

• Juice of 1 lemon

• 1 teaspoon chopped fresh dill

• 1 teaspoon chopped fresh parsley

• Salt and pepper to taste

Instructions:

1. Preheat oven to 375°F (190°C) and line a baking sheet with parchment paper.

2. Place salmon fillets on the prepared baking sheet.

3. In a small bowl, mix together olive oil, minced garlic, lemon zest, lemon juice, chopped dill, chopped parsley, salt, and pepper.

4. Spoon the mixture over each salmon fillet, spreading it evenly.

5. Bake for 12-15 minutes until the salmon is cooked through and flakes easily with a fork.

6. Serve the baked lemon herb salmon hot.

Greek Quinoa Salad

Ingredients:

• 2 cups cooked quinoa

• 1 cucumber (diced)

• 1 cup cherry tomatoes (halved)

• 1/2 cup Kalamata olives (pitted and halved)

• 1/4 cup red onion (finely chopped)

• 1/2 cup crumbled feta cheese

• 2 tablespoons chopped fresh parsley

For the dressing:

- 1/4 cup extra virgin olive oil

- 2 tablespoons red wine vinegar

- 1 teaspoon dried oregano

- Salt and pepper to taste

Instructions:

1. In a large bowl, combine cooked quinoa, diced cucumber, cherry tomatoes, Kalamata olives, chopped red onion, crumbled feta cheese, and chopped parsley.

2. In a small bowl, whisk together extra virgin olive oil, red wine vinegar, dried oregano, salt, and pepper to make the dressing.

3. Drizzle the dressing over the salad and toss gently to coat.

4. Serve the Greek quinoa salad chilled or at room temperature.

## Veggie Stir-Fry with Tofu

Ingredients:

- 1 block (14 oz) firm tofu (drained and cubed)

- 2 tablespoons low-sodium soy sauce

- 2 tablespoons olive oil

- 2 cloves garlic (minced)

- 1 teaspoon grated ginger

- Assorted vegetables (bell peppers, broccoli, snap peas)

- Cooked brown rice for serving

Instructions:

1. In a bowl, marinate tofu cubes in low-sodium soy sauce for about 10-15 minutes.

2. Heat olive oil in a large skillet or wok over medium-high heat. Add minced garlic and grated ginger, sauté for a minute.

3. Add marinated tofu cubes to the skillet and cook until lightly browned.

4. Add assorted vegetables to the skillet and stir-fry until tender-crisp.

5. Serve the tofu and vegetable stir-fry over cooked brown rice.

Ingredients:

- 1 pound ground turkey

- 2 tablespoons olive oil

- 1/2 onion (chopped)

- 2 cloves garlic (minced)

- 1 bell pepper (diced)

- 1 cup shredded carrots

- 1/2 cup water chestnuts (chopped)

- 2 tablespoons low-sodium soy sauce

- 1 tablespoon hoisin sauce

- Lettuce leaves for wrapping (butter lettuce or iceberg lettuce)

Instructions:

1. Heat olive oil in a skillet over medium heat. Add chopped onion and minced garlic, sauté until fragrant.

2. Add ground turkey to the skillet and cook until browned.

3. Stir in diced bell pepper, shredded carrots, and chopped water chestnuts. Cook for a few minutes until vegetables soften.

4. Add low-sodium soy sauce and hoisin sauce, stir to combine.

5. Spoon the turkey and veggie mixture onto lettuce leaves, wrap them up, and secure with toothpicks if needed.

6. Serve the turkey and veggie lettuce wraps as a healthy lunch option.

Mediterranean Quinoa Salad

Ingredients:

• 2 cups cooked quinoa

• 1 cucumber (diced)

• 1 cup cherry tomatoes (halved)

• 1/2 cup Kalamata olives (pitted and halved)

• 1/4 cup red onion (finely chopped)

• 1/2 cup crumbled feta cheese

• 2 tablespoons chopped fresh parsley

For the dressing:

- 1/4 cup extra virgin olive oil

- 2 tablespoons lemon juice

- 1 teaspoon dried oregano

- Salt and pepper to taste

Instructions:

1. In a large bowl, combine cooked quinoa, diced cucumber, cherry tomatoes, Kalamata olives, chopped red onion, crumbled feta cheese, and chopped parsley.

2. In a small bowl, whisk together extra virgin olive oil, lemon juice, dried oregano, salt, and pepper to make the dressing.

3. Drizzle the dressing over the salad and toss gently to coat.

4. Serve the Mediterranean quinoa salad chilled or at room temperature.


Lemon Garlic Chicken and Vegetable Skewers

Ingredients:

- 1-pound boneless, skinless chicken breasts (cut into cubes)

- 1 zucchini (sliced)

- 1 bell pepper (cut into chunks)

- 1 red onion (cut into chunks)

- 2 tablespoons olive oil

- 2 cloves garlic (minced)

- Zest of 1 lemon

- Juice of 1 lemon

- Salt and pepper to taste

Instructions:

1. Preheat grill or grill pan over medium-high heat.

2. Thread chicken cubes, zucchini slices, bell pepper chunks, and red onion onto skewers.

3. In a bowl, mix together olive oil, minced garlic, lemon zest, lemon juice, salt, and pepper.

4. Brush the marinade over the skewers, coating them evenly.

5. Grill the skewers for about 8-10 minutes, turning occasionally until chicken is cooked through and vegetables are tender.

6. Serve the lemon garlic chicken and vegetable skewers hot.

Ingredients:

- 1 pie crust (store-bought or homemade)

- 1 tablespoon olive oil

- 1 onion (chopped)

- 2 cups fresh spinach leaves

- 1 cup sliced mushrooms

- 4 eggs

- 1 cup milk (or unsweetened almond milk)

- 1/2 cup shredded cheese (such as mozzarella or cheddar)

- Salt and pepper to taste

Instructions:

1. Preheat oven to 375°F (190°C) and place the pie crust in a pie dish.

2. Heat olive oil in a skillet over medium heat. Add chopped onion and sauté until translucent.

3. Add spinach leaves and sliced mushrooms to the skillet. Cook until spinach wilts and mushrooms release their moisture.

4. Spread the cooked vegetables evenly over the pie crust.

5. In a bowl, whisk together eggs, milk, shredded cheese, salt, and pepper.

6. Pour the egg mixture over the vegetables in the pie crust. Bake for 35-40 minutes until the quiche is set and the crust is golden brown.

7. Let it cool for a few minutes before slicing.

Tofu and Vegetable Stir-Fry

Ingredients:

- 1 block (14 oz) firm tofu (drained and cubed)

- 2 tablespoons low-sodium soy sauce

- 2 tablespoons cornstarch

- 2 tablespoons olive oil

- 2 cloves garlic (minced)

- 1 teaspoon grated ginger

- Assorted vegetables (broccoli, bell peppers, snow peas)

- Cooked brown rice for serving

Instructions:

1. In a bowl, marinate tofu cubes in low-sodium soy sauce and cornstarch for about 10 minutes.

2. Heat olive oil in a large skillet or wok over medium-high heat. Add minced garlic and grated ginger, sauté for a minute.

3. Add marinated tofu cubes to the skillet and cook until crispy.

4. Add assorted vegetables to the skillet and stir-fry until tender-crisp.

5. Serve the tofu and vegetable stir-fry over cooked brown rice.


Turkey and Spinach Stuffed Bell Peppers

Ingredients:

• 4 bell peppers (any color)

• 1 pound ground turkey

• 1 tablespoon olive oil

• 1 onion (chopped)

• 2 cloves garlic (minced)

• 2 cups fresh spinach leaves (chopped)

- 1 cup cooked quinoa

- 1 can (14 oz) diced tomatoes (with juices)

- Salt and pepper to taste

- Shredded cheese for topping (optional)

Instructions:

1. Preheat oven to 375°F (190°C). Cut the tops off the bell peppers and remove seeds.

2. In a skillet, heat olive oil over medium heat. Add chopped onion and minced garlic, sauté until fragrant.

3. Add ground turkey to the skillet and cook until browned. Stir in chopped spinach and cooked quinoa, cook until spinach wilts.

4. Add diced tomatoes (with juices), salt, and pepper. Cook for a few minutes.

5. Spoon the turkey and spinach mixture into each bell pepper.

6. Optionally, sprinkle shredded cheese on top of each stuffed pepper.

7. Place the stuffed peppers in a baking dish and bake for 25-30 minutes until peppers are tender.

Tomato-Poached Cod with Fresh Herbs

Ingredients:

- 2 tablespoons extra-virgin olive oil

- 1 shallot, thinly sliced

- Kosher salt and freshly ground black pepper

- 1 garlic clove, thinly sliced

- ½ teaspoon crushed red pepper flakes, or more, as desired

- Two 14-ounce cans crushed tomatoes and their liquid

- 1 cup low-sodium vegetable stock (or water)

- Four 5-ounce cod fillets

- 1 cup parsley or basil leaves and fine stems, roughly chopped or torn, for sprinkling

- Toasted crusty bread, for serving

Instructions:

1. Heat the oil in a wide, shallow skillet over medium heat until shimmering. Add the shallot and salt, stirring until softened, about 3 minutes. Add the garlic and pepper flakes, stirring until fragrant, about 30 seconds more.

2. Pour in the tomatoes and stock and raise the heat to bring the mixture to a boil. Lower the heat to a simmer, stirring occasionally, and season with salt and pepper. Let it cook until the tomatoes lose their tinned taste and the liquid reduces slightly, 8 to 10 minutes

3. Season the fish with salt and pepper and add to the sauce, adjusting the heat to maintain a gentle simmer. Cook, spooning the sauce over the fillets occasionally, until the fish is opaque and easily flakes when touched, about 5 minutes. If they are not fully submerged, turn them over halfway. (Thick fillets will take a little longer.)

4. Divide the fish between serving bowls and spoon the tomato sauce on top. Finish with pepper and parsley and serve with the bread for dipping.

5. NOTE: To add more heat to the dish, you can stir in ½ to 1 tablespoon harissa when adding the shallots and garlic.

Sweet Potato Noodle Enchilada Stir-Fry

Ingredients:

• 1.5 pounds sweet potatoes spiralize with B blade

• 1 tablespoon olive oil

• 1 yellow onion chopped

- 2 cloves garlic minced

- 1 teaspoon ground cumin

- 1 14.5 oz can fire-roasted tomatoes with green chilies (don't drain) this is spicy!

- 1 15 oz can black beans, drained and rinsed (or cook your own from scratch)

- 1 teaspoon salt

- Chopped fresh cilantro for garnish

- Feta cheese optional

Instructions:

1. Peel and slice the ends off of the sweet potatoes, then create "noodles" by using the B blade on the Inspiralizer. Set them aside.

2. Heat the olive oil in a deep skillet or Dutch oven over medium heat, and sauté the onion until it starts to soften, about 5 minutes. Add in the minced garlic and cumin, and stir until fragrant, about 1 minute.

3. Add in the sweet potato noodles, fire-roasted tomatoes (including the juice), black beans, and salt, and stir well. The liquid from the tomatoes should start simmering. Once you hear the simmer, lower the heat and cover the pan with a lid for 10 minutes to let the sweet potatoes soften.

4. Remove the lid and stir well, and test the sweet potatoes with a fork to see if they are tender enough to your liking. If there is a lot of liquid at the bottom of the pan, simply raise the heat and stir well, so that it simmers away and evaporates.

5. Adjust any seasoning to taste, and serve warm with a sprinkling of fresh cilantro, and a sprinkling of cheese, if desired.

6. Leftovers can be stored in the fridge for up to 5 days. To reheat, simply dump the leftovers in a skillet over medium heat again and stir until warm.

Slow-Cooker Pasta e Fagioli Soup

Ingredients:

• One 28-ounce can crushed tomatoes

• 1 sweet onion, diced

• 1½ cups dried white beans, soaked in cool water overnight and drained

• 2 carrots, peeled and sliced

• 2 stalks celery, sliced

• 4 garlic cloves, minced

- 1 Parmesan rind

- ½ cup dry white wine

- 4 cups low-sodium chicken or vegetable broth

- Large pinch crushed red pepper flakes

- 1 bay leaf

- 3 sprigs fresh thyme

- 2 sprigs fresh rosemary

- Kosher salt and freshly ground black pepper

- 1¼ cup short pasta (such as ditalini)

- 1 bunch lacinato kale, roughly torn

- ⅓ cup chopped fresh parsley

- Parmesan cheese, for serving

Instructions:

1. Place the tomatoes, onion, beans carrots, celery, garlic, Parmesan rind, white wine and broth in the bowl of a slow cooker.

2. Add the red pepper flakes, bay leaf, thyme and rosemary. Turn the slow cooker on low and cook until the beans are tender, about 7 hours.

3. Season the soup with salt and pepper. Stir in the pasta and the kale. Turn the slow cooker to high and cook until the pasta is tender, about 30 minutes.

4. Stir in the parsley just before serving and garnish with the Parmesan.

Corn and Tomato Salad with Feta and Lime

Ingredients:

• Extra-virgin olive oil, as needed

• 4 cups fresh corn (from about 7 small ears of corn)

• Kosher salt and freshly ground black pepper

• ½ cup cherry tomatoes, halved

• 4 ounces feta cheese, cubed

• Juice of one lime

• 1 bunch fresh cilantro, roughly chopped

Instructions:

1. In a large skillet, heat a few tablespoons olive oil over medium heat. Add the corn, and season with salt and pepper. Cook, stirring occasionally, until the corn starts to soften, about 5 minutes. Add the cherry tomatoes and cook, stirring

occasionally, until they release their juices, about 5 minutes more.

2. Remove the skillet from the heat and stir in the feta cheese. Taste and adjust the seasoning with salt and pepper as needed. Stir in the cilantro and lime juice, and transfer to a serving bowl. Serve warm or at room temperature.

Roasted Brussels Sprouts Quinoa

Ingredients:

• 6 large carrots, peeled and cut into bite-size pieces

• 1 pound Brussels sprouts, halved

• 1 large red onion, sliced

• 2 tablespoons extra-virgin olive oil

• Kosher salt and freshly ground pepper

• 2 cups chicken stock

• 1 cup quinoa, rinsed

• 2 teaspoons fresh thyme

Instructions:

1. Preheat the oven to 450°F. On a baking sheet, toss the carrots, Brussels sprouts and red onion with the olive oil; season with salt and pepper.

2. Roast the vegetables until fork-tender, 15 to 20 minutes.

3. In a large microwave-safe bowl, combine the chicken stock, quinoa and thyme; season with salt and pepper. Cover the bowl tightly with plastic wrap and microwave it on high for 6 minutes. If there's a lot of liquid remaining, microwave until it's absorbed, about 3 more minutes.

4. Transfer the vegetables and any remaining olive oil from the baking sheet to the bowl and stir to combine; season with salt and pepper to taste.


Summer Millet Salad

Ingredients:

• 1 cup millet

• 2¼ cups water or vegetable broth

• 4 scallions, chopped

• 1 pint cherry tomatoes, quartered

- 1¼ cups cubed Havarti cheese

- 1 cup parsley leaves

- 1 lemon, zested and juiced

- ⅓ cup olive oil

- Kosher salt and freshly ground black pepper

Instructions:

1. In a medium saucepan, combine the millet with the water or broth. Bring to a simmer over medium heat. Cover the pot and reduce the heat to low.

2. Simmer until the liquid is absorbed and the millet is fluffy, 12 to 15 minutes. Drain the millet in a strainer and cool to room temperature.

3. In a large bowl, toss the cooled millet with the scallions, tomatoes, cheese, parsley and lemon zest.

4. Pour the lemon juice and olive oil over the mixture and toss to coat. Season with salt and pepper to taste. Reserve in an airtight container in the refrigerator until ready to serve (it will keep for up to five days).

Ingredients:

• 14 ounces waxy new potatoes, halved

• 2 tablespoons olive oil, divided

• 4 skin-on chicken thighs

• 1½ teaspoons dried oregano

• 1½ teaspoons dried thyme

• 7 ounces feta, crumbled

• ⅔ cup pitted Kalamata olives

• 5½ ounces cherry tomatoes

• 1 tablespoon red wine vinegar

• Kosher salt and freshly ground black pepper

• Fresh oregano leaves and lemon wedges, for serving

Instructions:

1. Preheat the oven to 400°F. Line a baking dish with parchment paper or aluminum foil.

2. In a large bowl, toss the potatoes with 1 tablespoon of the olive oil and some salt, then spread onto the lined baking dish.

Season the chicken thighs with salt and pepper, rub on the remaining olive oil and top with the dried herbs.

3. Nestle the chicken on top of the potatoes, close up the parchment or foil into a tight packet and transfer to the oven for 40 minutes.

4. Carefully open up the packet, add in the crumbled feta, olives, cherry tomatoes and red wine vinegar and return to the oven, uncovered, until the potatoes are tender and the chicken is cooked through, 35 to 40 minutes. (Test the doneness by inserting a skewer into each thigh and checking the juices run clear.) Remove from the oven and serve fresh oregano leaves and lemon wedges.

Spiced Lamb Meatball and Escarole Soup

Ingredients:

- 1¼ pounds ground lamb

- 3 large garlic cloves, minced

- 1 tablespoon ground coriander

- 1 tablespoon ground cumin

- 2 teaspoons dried oregano

- 2 teaspoons ground turmeric

- ½ teaspoon paprika

- 2¾ teaspoons kosher salt, plus more as needed

- 1¼ teaspoons freshly ground black pepper

- 2 tablespoons extra-virgin olive oil

- 2 large onions, sliced

- ¼ cup tomato paste

- 8 cups broth (homemade or high-quality store-bought)

- 1 large head escarole, torn into 2-inch pieces

- 1½ cups cooked gigante or cannellini beans or one 15.5-ounce can, drained and rinsed

- Flaky sea salt (optional)

- Lemon wedges, for serving

Instructions:

1. MAKE THE MEATBALLS: In a large bowl, mix the lamb, garlic, coriander, cumin, oregano, turmeric, paprika, 1 teaspoon of the salt and 1 teaspoon of the pepper. Pinch off 1 ounce (2 scant tablespoons) of the lamb mixture at a time and gently roll it into a ball with your hands. Place on a plate and repeat with the remaining lamb mixture.

2. In a large pot, heat the oil over medium-high heat. Add the meatballs and cook until golden brown and crispy on all sides, 7 to 9 minutes. Transfer to a plate. Pour off 3 tablespoons of the fat from the pan.

3. MAKE THE SOUP: Add the onions, ¼ teaspoon of the salt and the remaining ¼ teaspoon pepper to the fat remaining in the pot. Cook over medium-high heat, stirring often, until the onions are golden and everything is softened, 8 to 10 minutes. Add the tomato paste and cook, stirring continuously, for about 1 minute to cook off the raw tomato flavor. Add the broth and 1 teaspoon salt and bring to a boil.

4. Add the escarole, beans, meatballs, and remaining ¼ teaspoon salt and return the soup to a simmer. Cook until the escarole has wilted and the meatballs have cooked through, 4 to 6 minutes more. Taste and season with salt and pepper.

5. Ladle into bowls, sprinkle with flaky sea salt (if you want), and serve with a lemon wedge alongside.


Easy 3 Cup Chicken with Zucchini

Ingredients:

• 1/3 cup low sodium soy sauce

• 1/3 cup rice vinegar

• 4 tablespoons sesame oil

- 1 1/2 pounds boneless skinless chicken breasts or thighs, cut in to 2-3 inch pieces

- 1-inch fresh ginger, thinly sliced

- 3 cloves garlic, thinly sliced

- 1 teaspoon chili flakes

- 1 zucchini, chopped

- 1 bell pepper, sliced

- 1 cup fresh basil

- rice for serving

Instructions

1. In a small bowl, combine the soy sauce, rice vinegar, and 2 tablespoons sesame oil.

2. Heat a large skillet over medium high heat and add the remaining 2 tablespoons sesame oil. When the oil shimmers, add the chicken and cook, stirring occasionally until the chicken is cooked through, about 8-10 minutes. Add the ginger and garlic, and cook another minute more.

3. Pour in the soy sauce/rice vinegar mixture and toss in the zucchini and bell pepper. Cook until the sauce thickens and coats the chicken, about 5-10 minutes.

4. Remove the skillet from the stove and stir in the basil. Serve over rice. Enjoy!

Pan-Fried Cod with Orange and Swiss Chard

Ingredients:

• Four 6-ounce cod fillets

• Salt and freshly ground black pepper

• 1 cup all-purpose flour

• ½ teaspoon cayenne pepper

• 4 tablespoons extra-virgin olive oil

• 1 red onion, thinly sliced

• 1 orange, halved and thinly sliced

• ¼ cup chopped fresh parsley, plus more for garnish

• 2½ cups chopped Swiss chard

• Orange wedges, for serving

Instructions:

1. Season each cod fillet on both sides with salt and pepper. Put the flour in a large bowl and stir in the cayenne pepper. Dredge each piece of cod thoroughly in the flour.

2. In a large sauté pan, heat the olive oil over medium heat. Add the cod and pan-fry until browned and fully cooked, about 3 to 4 minutes on each side.

3. Remove the cod from the pan and drain all but 1 tablespoon of oil. Add the onion and orange, and sauté until the onion is tender, 4 to 5 minutes. Stir in the parsley and Swiss chard, and cook until tender, 3 to 4 minutes more.

4. Transfer each piece of cod to a plate and divide the onion, orange and Swiss chard mixture evenly among the plates. Garnish with more parsley and orange wedges. Serve immediately.


Crispy Za'atar Chicken and Cauliflower

Ingredients:

• 2 tablespoons (30ml) melted ghee or clarified butter

• 3 tablespoons (23g) za'atar

• 1 tablespoons (15ml) fresh lemon juice

- 1½ tsp (9g) kosher salt

- 1 head cauliflower, cut into florets (about 4 cups or 400g)

- 1 red onion, cut into 1-inch wedges

- 3 garlic heads, tops trimmed

- 2 lemons, halved

- 2 pounds (905g) bone-in, skin-on chicken thighs (about 4 large thighs)

Instructions:

1. Preheat the oven to 425°F and line a rimmed baking sheet with foil.

2. In a small bowl, combine the melted ghee, za'atar, lemon juice and salt. Place the cauliflower, onion, garlic heads, halved lemons and chicken on the prepared baking sheet. Add the seasoning mixture and toss until evenly coated. Arrange everything into a single layer on the baking sheet.

3. Bake until the chicken is cooked, 40 to 45 minutes, then broil on high until the skin is crispy, about 1 minute. Squeeze the roasted garlic cloves out of the heads and sprinkle over the chicken, then serve.

4. NOTE: The chicken can be seasoned the night before and stored in a resealable plastic bag in the refrigerator until ready to cook, to get your dinner on the table even faster.

Ingredients:

- 1 cup freekeh (cracked or whole)

- 3 tablespoons extra-virgin olive oil, plus more for drizzling

- 1 large onion, diced

- 1 medium kohlrabi, rind and tough outer membranes peeled off, diced

- 2 medium carrots, diced

- 1 teaspoon kosher salt, plus more for seasoning

- ½ teaspoon freshly ground black pepper, plus more for seasoning

- 3 garlic cloves, minced

- 8 cups vegetable or chicken broth, plus more if needed

- 2 medium zucchini, diced

- 1 Parmesan rind or 1 tablespoon nutritional yeast (optional)

- 2 teaspoons chopped fresh za'atar or oregano

- ¼ teaspoon cayenne pepper, or more to taste

• Chopped fresh herbs (za'atar, parsley, chives or scallions), for garnish

Instructions:

1. Place the freekeh in a medium bowl, cover with cold water and set aside.

2. Heat the olive oil in a large 4- or 5-quart saucepan over medium heat. Add the onion and cook, stirring, until softened, 6 to 8 minutes. Add the kohlrabi and carrots and cook, stirring, until the vegetables begin to soften, about 5 minutes; season generously with salt and black pepper. Add the garlic and cook about 1 minute more.

3. Drain the freekeh, rinse it with cold water and add it to the saucepan. Add the broth, zucchini, Parmesan rind (if using), za'atar, salt and the cayenne. Bring to a boil, then reduce the heat and simmer uncovered until the soup is thickened, 25 to 30 minutes (or a few minutes longer if you're using whole freekeh instead of cracked freekeh).

4. Remove the Parmesan rind, season with more salt and black pepper to taste, divide among bowls, garnish with herbs and drizzle with olive oil.

# Pasta alla Norma with Eggplant, Basil & Pecorino

Ingredients:

- 4 tablespoons extra-virgin olive oil

- 1 large eggplant, sliced into 1-inch strips

- Kosher salt and freshly ground black pepper

- 1 sweet onion, thinly sliced

- 3 garlic cloves, peeled and crushed

- One 28-ounce can crushed tomatoes

- 1 teaspoon crushed red pepper flakes

- ¾ teaspoon dried oregano

- 1 pound bite-size dry pasta, like rigatoni or macaroni

- ¼ cup chopped fresh parsley

- ¼ cup chopped fresh basil

- ½ cup grated pecorino or ricotta salata cheese

Instructions:

1. In a large sauté pan, heat the olive oil over medium heat. Add the eggplant in batches and cook on all sides until golden

brown. Remove the eggplant from the pan and set aside on a large plate. Season to taste with salt and pepper.

2. To the same pan, add the onion and sauté until tender, about 4 minutes. Add the garlic and sauté until fragrant, about 1 minute more.

3. Stir in the tomatoes and bring to a simmer. Add the red pepper flakes and oregano, and season with salt and pepper. Simmer until the flavor of the sauce develops and concentrates slightly, 15 to 20 minutes.

4. While the sauce simmers, bring a large pot of salted water to a boil over high heat. Add the pasta and cook according to the instructions on the package. Drain well.

5. Add the pasta and eggplant to the sauce; toss to coat. Add the parsley, basil and pecorino or ricotta salata, and toss well to combine.

Greek Chicken and Rice Skillet

Ingredients:

• 6 chicken thighs

• Kosher salt and freshly ground black pepper

• 1 teaspoon dried oregano

- 1 teaspoon garlic powder

- 3 lemons

- 2 tablespoons extra-virgin olive oil

- ½ red onion, minced

- 2 garlic cloves, minced

- 1 cup long-grain rice

- 2½ cups chicken broth

- 1 tablespoon chopped fresh oregano, plus more for garnishing

- 1 cup green olives

- ½ cup crumbled feta cheese

- ⅓ cup fresh chopped fresh parsley

Instructions:

1. Preheat the oven to 375°F. Season the chicken thighs with salt and pepper. In a small bowl, stir together the dried oregano, garlic powder and the zest of 1 lemon. Rub the mixture evenly over the chicken.

2. Heat the olive oil in a large oven-safe skillet over medium heat. Add the chicken, skin side down, and sear until the

chicken is well browned, 7 to 9 minutes. Remove to a plate and reserve.

3. Add the onion and garlic to the skillet and sauté until translucent, about 5 minutes. Stir in the rice and sauté for 1 minute; season with salt.

4. Add the chicken broth and bring the mixture to a simmer. Stir in the fresh oregano and the juice of the zested lemon. Slice the remaining 2 lemons and set aside.

5. Nestle the chicken, skin side up, into the rice mixture. Transfer the skillet to the oven and cook until the rice has absorbed all of the liquid and the chicken is fully cooked, 20 to 25 minutes.

6. Turn on the broiler and arrange the lemon slices over the chicken. Broil the skillet until the lemons are lightly charred and the chicken skin is very crisp, about 3 minutes.

7. Add the olives and feta to the skillet, garnish with fresh parsley and serve immediately.

Ingredients:

- ¼ cup honey

- ¼ cup tahini

- 3 tablespoons fresh lemon juice, plus 1 lemon, halved

- 2 tablespoons extra-virgin olive oil

- Pinch of kosher salt and freshly ground black pepper

- 2 pounds salmon fillets

- One 15-ounce can chickpeas, rinsed and drained

- 1 cup couscous

- ¼ cup chopped fresh parsley, plus more for garnish

- ¼ cup golden raisins, plus more for garnish

- ⅛ teaspoon crushed red pepper flakes

- 1¼ cups vegetable or chicken stock (store-bought or homemade)

- ⅓ cup toasted chopped almonds

- 1 tablespoon za'atar

• Labne or Greek yogurt, for serving

Instructions:

1. Preheat the oven to 400°F.

2. In a small bowl, whisk together the honey, tahini, lemon juice, olive oil, salt and pepper. Using a pastry brush or spoon, evenly coat the salmon fillets with the sauce on all sides. Place the fillets in the center of a sheet pan along with the halved lemon, cut side up, and roast for 10 minutes.

3. After 10 minutes, carefully slide the sheet pan out of the oven and add the chickpeas, couscous, chopped parsley, raisins, pepper flakes in an even layer surrounding the salmon and lemon. Pour the stock over the couscous mixture, and return to the oven. Cook until the salmon is medium-rare and flakes easily with a fork and the couscous is cooked through and tender, 6 to 8 minutes.

4. To serve, garnish with more parsley and raisins and the za'atar and almonds. Serve with labne or Greek yogurt on the side.

Pasta Puttanesca

Ingredients:

• Extra-virgin olive oil, as needed

• 1 garlic clove, crushed

• 1 shallot, diced

• One 2-ounce (45g) tin anchovies, drained

• One 14-ounce (400g) can whole peeled tomatoes

• 2 teaspoons red wine vinegar

• 2½ cups (200g) penne (or any other kind of dried pasta)

• 10 Niçoise olives, pitted

• 1 cup (100g) halved cherry tomatoes

• Two 5-ounce (140g) tins tuna (preferred pole & line caught and MSC certified) in olive oil, drained

• Kosher salt and freshly ground black pepper, as needed

• ½ bunch of basil, leaves only

Instructions:

1. Heat a generous splash of olive oil in a skillet over medium-high heat, and cook the garlic and shallot until soft, about 3

minutes. Add the anchovy fillets and let them "melt" while stirring continuously, about 2 minutes.

2. Add the tomatoes and vinegar and let the mixture simmer with a lid on, about 4 minutes, then crush the mixture with a potato masher or the back of a wooden spoon.

3. Meanwhile, bring a large pot of generously salted water to a boil over medium-high heat. Cook the pasta to al dente or according to the package directions.

4. Add the olives and cherry tomatoes to the shallot-tomato mixture and gently simmer over low heat, about 3 minutes. Fold in the drained tuna, and heat through for about 2 minutes, then season with pepper and salt if needed.

5. Drain the pasta in a colander, then carefully stir the pasta into the tomato sauce. Divide the pasta puttanesca between two plates, drizzle with olive oil and serve garnished with basil.

Fall Roasted Vegetable and Lentil Salad with Pine Nut Cream

Ingredients:

PINE NUT CREAM

- ½ cup pine nuts

- ¼ cup cilantro leaves

- 3 to 4 tablespoons water

- 3 tablespoons freshly squeezed lemon juice

- 1 tablespoon olive oil

- ¾ teaspoons kosher salt

ROASTED VEGETABLE AND LENTIL SALAD

- 3 tablespoons extra-virgin olive oil, plus more for drizzling

- 1 tablespoon whole-grain mustard

- 1½ teaspoons kosher salt

- 1 teaspoon coriander seeds (optional)

- 1 teaspoon dried thyme

- ½ teaspoon freshly ground black pepper

- 1 medium delicata squash, cut in half lengthwise then cut into ½-inch half circles (you can remove seeds or leave them)

- 1 pound baby yellow potatoes, cut in half

- 3 medium yellow beets — stems removed, peeled and cut into 1-inch pieces

- 1½ cups cooked lentils

Instructions:

1. MAKE THE PINE NUT CREAM: In a blender, combine the pine nuts, cilantro, water, lemon juice, olive oil and salt, and puree until smooth and a bit chunky. Set aside.

2. MAKE THE SALAD: Preheat the oven to 400°F. In a small bowl, whisk together the olive oil, mustard, salt, coriander seeds (if using), thyme and black pepper. Arrange the squash, potatoes and beets on a baking sheet and drizzle the olive oil mixture on top, tossing to coat. Make sure the vegetables are not overlapping and are spread out so they caramelize evenly.

3. Bake the vegetables until they are deeply caramelized, 25 to 30 minutes. If you left the squash seeds on, make sure these are deeply browned too — they will be crunchy and chewy when you bite into them.

4. To assemble the salad, spread some of the pine nut cream on a large platter. Top with the roasted vegetables and cooked lentils. Drizzle with more pine nut cream and a bit of olive oil before serving.

5. NOTE: To cook lentils, add 1 cup lentils to 3 cups salted boiling water. Cook for 15 minutes, then drain and set aside. The lentils should be al dente.

Sheet Pan Curried Butternut Squash Soup

Ingredients:

• 1 medium butternut squash—peeled, seeded and cubed (about 7 cups)

• Extra-virgin olive oil, as needed

• Kosher salt and freshly ground black pepper

• 1 small yellow onion, peeled and quartered

• 1 head garlic, halved crosswise

• 2 teaspoons curry powder, plus more as needed

• 1 teaspoon chili powder, plus more as needed

• ¼ teaspoon cayenne, plus more as needed

• ¼ teaspoon ground cinnamon

• 4 cups chicken stock

• ½ cup coconut milk (optional)

Instructions:

1. Preheat oven to 425°F.

2. On an unlined rimmed baking sheet, drizzle the squash, onion and garlic with olive oil, then toss with the curry powder,

chili powder, cayenne and cinnamon. Season generously with salt and pepper.

3. Transfer to the oven and roast until tender and golden brown, 35 to 45 minutes.

4. Transfer the roasted vegetables to a high-speed blender (or use an immersion blender) and squeeze the roasted garlic out of its peel. Puree with the chicken stock until completely smooth. Taste and adjust the seasoning as needed.

5. Transfer to a Dutch oven or large saucepan and stir in the coconut milk, if using. Warm as needed before serving.


Salmon with Pesto and Blistered Tomatoes

Ingredients:

• 1-pound mixed cherry tomatoes

• 3 garlic cloves, minced

• Kosher salt and freshly ground black pepper

• 3 tablespoons extra-virgin olive oil

• 1 large (1 to 1½ pounds) center-cut salmon fillet or 4 small fillets (3 to 4 ounces each)

• 1 cup basil pesto (store-bought or homemade)

Instructions:

1. Preheat the oven to 425°F. Line a baking sheet with parchment paper.

2. On the baking sheet, toss together the cherry tomatoes, garlic and a sprinkle of salt and pepper. Bake until the tomatoes have burst and are slightly browned, 15 to 16 minutes.

3. Line a separate baking sheet with parchment paper for the salmon. Brush a light coat of olive oil onto the fillet(s) and season with salt and pepper.

4. Bake for 10 minutes, then spoon 1 to 2 tablespoons of the pesto evenly over the salmon. Bake until the salmon flakes off easily when prodded with a fork, about 3 minutes more.

5. Gently transfer the salmon to a serving platter and top with the burst tomatoes.

6. NOTE: If you don't love salmon, you can replace it with cod or halibut.

Ingredients:

## SEED-NUT CRUNCH

- 1 teaspoon extra-virgin olive oil

- 3 tablespoons pumpkin seeds

- 2 tablespoons pine nuts

- 1 teaspoon granulated sugar

- 1 teaspoon white miso

- ½ teaspoon harissa powder or paprika

- Small pinch kosher salt

## SOUP

- 3 tablespoons extra-virgin olive oil, plus more for drizzling

- 1 medium yellow onion, peeled and cut into medium pieces

- 2 garlic cloves, peeled and crushed

- 1 medium fennel bulb, core removed and cut into a medium dice

- 1½ pounds (7 to 8 medium) carrots, scrubbed and cut into medium pieces

- 1 teaspoon kosher salt

- 3 tablespoons white miso

- 4 cups water

Instructions:

1. MAKE THE CRUNCH: Heat a small skillet over medium heat. Add the olive oil, pumpkin seeds and pine nuts. Stir and cook until they begin to toast and smell nutty, about 1 minute.

2. Add the sugar, miso, harissa powder and salt, and continue cooking while stirring constantly until the sugar and miso melt and everything caramelizes, about 1 minute. Be careful not to burn the pumpkin seeds and pine nuts. Immediately transfer to a plate and spread out the mixture to cool. Store in an airtight container for up to a week.

3. MAKE THE SOUP: Heat a large (7-quart) Dutch oven or stock pot over medium-high heat. Add the olive oil, onion, garlic, fennel, carrot and salt. Cook the vegetables, stirring occasionally, until they begin to caramelize, 8 to 10 minutes.

4. Add the miso and continue cooking, stirring constantly, until caramelized, about 1 minute more. The vegetables should have a slightly caramelized color — this will give the soup depth of flavor.

5. Add the water and bring to a simmer, then reduce the heat to medium-low, cover the pot and cook until the vegetables are

tender, 15 to 20 minutes. Using an immersion blender or high-speed blender, puree the soup. Taste and adjust the salt if needed. Serve the soup with the seed-nut crunch and a drizzle of olive oil.

Sheet-Pan Chicken Thighs with Brussels Sprouts & Gnocchi

Ingredients:

- 4 tablespoons extra-virgin olive oil, divided

- 2 tablespoons chopped fresh oregano, divided

- 2 large cloves garlic, minced, divided

- ½ teaspoon ground pepper, divided

- ¼ teaspoon salt, divided

- 1-pound Brussels sprouts, trimmed and quartered

- 1 (16 ounce) package shelf-stable gnocchi

- 1 cup sliced red onion

- 4 boneless, skinless chicken thighs, trimmed

- 1 cup halved cherry tomatoes

- 1 tablespoon red-wine vinegar

Instructions:

1. Preheat oven to 450 degrees F.

2. Stir 2 tablespoons oil, 1 tablespoon oregano, half the garlic, 1/4 teaspoon pepper and 1/8 teaspoon salt together in a large bowl. Add Brussels sprouts, gnocchi and onion; toss to coat. Spread on a large rimmed baking sheet.

3. Stir 1 tablespoon oil, the remaining 1 tablespoon oregano, the remaining garlic and the remaining 1/4 teaspoon pepper and 1/8 teaspoon salt in the large bowl. Add chicken and toss to coat. Nestle the chicken into the vegetable mixture. Roast for 10 minutes.

4. Remove from the oven and add the tomatoes; stir to combine. Continue roasting until the Brussels sprouts are tender and the chicken is just cooked through, about 10 minutes more. Stir vinegar and the remaining 1 tablespoon oil into the vegetable mixture.


Mushroom & Tofu Stir-Fry

Ingredients:

• 4 tablespoons peanut oil or canola oil, divided

• 1-pound mixed mushrooms, sliced

• 1 medium red bell pepper, diced

- 1 bunch scallions, trimmed and cut into 2-inch pieces

- 1 tablespoon grated fresh ginger

- 1 large clove garlic, grated

- 1 (8 ounce) container baked tofu or smoked tofu, diced

- 3 tablespoons oyster sauce or vegetarian oyster sauce

Instructions:

1. Heat 2 tablespoons oil in a large flat-bottom wok or cast-iron skillet over high heat. Add mushrooms and bell pepper; cook, stirring occasionally, until soft, about 4 minutes. Stir in scallions, ginger and garlic; cook for 30 seconds more. Transfer the vegetables to a bowl.

2. Add the remaining 2 tablespoons oil and tofu to the pan. Cook, turning once, until browned, 3 to 4 minutes. Stir in the vegetables and oyster sauce. Cook, stirring, until hot, about 1 minute.

Cod and Asparagus Bake

Ingredients:

- 4 cod fillets (4 ounces each)

- 1-pound fresh thin asparagus, trimmed

- 1-pint cherry tomatoes, halved

- 2 tablespoons lemon juice

- 1-1/2 teaspoons grated lemon zest

- 1/4 cup grated Romano cheese

Instructions:

1. Preheat oven to 375°. Place cod and asparagus in a 15x10x1-in. baking pan brushed with oil. Add tomatoes, cut sides down. Brush fish with lemon juice; sprinkle with lemon zest. Sprinkle fish and vegetables with Romano cheese. Bake until fish just begins to flake easily with a fork, about 12 minutes.

2. Remove pan from oven; preheat broiler. Broil cod mixture 3-4 in. from heat until vegetables are lightly browned, 2-3 minutes.

Salmon with Spinach and White Beans

Ingredients:

- 4 salmon fillets (4 ounces each)

- 2 teaspoons plus 1 tablespoon olive oil, divided

- 1 teaspoon seafood seasoning

- 1 garlic clove, minced

- 1 can (15 ounces) cannellini beans, rinsed and drained

- 1/4 teaspoon salt

- 1/4 teaspoon pepper

- 1 package (8 ounces) fresh spinach

- Lemon wedges

Instructions:

1. Preheat broiler. Rub fillets with 2 teaspoons oil; sprinkle with seafood seasoning. Place on a greased rack of a broiler pan. Broil 5-6 in. from heat 6-8 minutes or until fish just begins to flake easily with a fork.

2. Meanwhile, in a large skillet, heat remaining oil over medium heat. Add garlic; cook 15-30 seconds or until fragrant. Add beans, salt and pepper, stirring to coat beans with garlic oil. Stir in spinach until wilted. Serve salmon with spinach mixture and lemon wedges.

Skillet Chicken with Olives

Ingredients:

- 4 boneless skinless chicken thighs (about 1 pound)

- 1 teaspoon dried rosemary, crushed

- 1/2 teaspoon pepper

- 1/4 teaspoon salt

- 1 tablespoon olive oil

- 1/2 cup pimiento-stuffed olives, coarsely chopped

- 1/4 cup white wine or chicken broth

- 1 tablespoon drained capers, optional

Instructions:

1. Sprinkle chicken with rosemary, pepper and salt. In a large skillet, heat oil over medium-high heat. Brown chicken on both sides.

2. Add olives, wine and, if desired, capers. Reduce heat; simmer, covered, 2-3 minutes or until a thermometer inserted in chicken reads 170°.

Mediterranean Pork and Orzo

Ingredients:

- 1-1/2 pounds pork tenderloin

- 1 teaspoon coarsely ground pepper

- 2 tablespoons olive oil

- 3 quarts water

- 1-1/4 cups uncooked orzo pasta

- 1/4 teaspoon salt

- 1 package (6 ounces) fresh baby spinach

- 1 cup grape tomatoes, halved

- 3/4 cup crumbled feta cheese

Instructions:

1. Rub pork with pepper; cut into 1-in. cubes. In a large nonstick skillet, heat oil over medium heat. Add pork; cook and stir until no longer pink, 8-10 minutes.

2. Meanwhile, in a Dutch oven, bring water to a boil. Stir in orzo and salt; cook, uncovered, 8 minutes. Stir in spinach; cook until orzo is tender and spinach is wilted, 45-60 seconds longer. Drain.

3. Add tomatoes to pork; heat through. Stir in orzo mixture and cheese.

# CHAPTER THREE

## DESSERT RECIPES

Berry Oatmeal Crumble Bars

Ingredients:

- 2 cups rolled oats

- 1 cup whole wheat flour

- 1/2 cup honey or maple syrup

- 1/2 cup coconut oil (melted)

- 1 teaspoon vanilla extract

- 2 cups mixed berries (strawberries, blueberries, raspberries)

- 2 tablespoons chia seeds

- 2 tablespoons lemon juice

- Zest of 1 lemon

Instructions:

1. Preheat oven to 350°F (175°C) and line a baking dish with parchment paper.

2. In a bowl, mix rolled oats, whole wheat flour, honey or maple syrup, melted coconut oil, and vanilla extract until crumbly.

3. Reserve half of the mixture and press the remaining mixture into the bottom of the baking dish to form a crust.

4. In another bowl, combine mixed berries, chia seeds, lemon juice, and lemon zest. Mash lightly with a fork.

5. Spread the berry mixture evenly over the crust. Sprinkle the reserved oat mixture on top of the berries.

6. Bake for 25-30 minutes until the top is golden brown.

7. Let it cool completely before slicing into bars.

## Dark Chocolate-Dipped Strawberries

Ingredients:

- Fresh strawberries

- Dark chocolate chips (70% cocoa or higher)

- Chopped nuts or shredded coconut for topping (optional)

Instructions:

1. Wash and pat dry the strawberries, leaving the stems intact.

2. In a microwave-safe bowl, melt the dark chocolate chips in 30-second intervals, stirring in between until smooth.

3. Dip each strawberry into the melted chocolate, coating about two-thirds of the berry.

4. Optional: Roll the chocolate-covered part in chopped nuts or shredded coconut.

5. Place the dipped strawberries on a parchment-lined tray and refrigerate for about 20-30 minutes until the chocolate hardens.

Banana-Oat Chocolate Chip Cookies

Ingredients:

• 2 ripe bananas (mashed)

• 1 1/2 cups rolled oats

• 1/4 cup dark chocolate chips

• 1/4 cup chopped nuts (walnuts or almonds)

• 1/2 teaspoon cinnamon

• 1/4 teaspoon nutmeg (optional)

Instructions:

1. Preheat oven to 350°F (175°C) and line a baking sheet with parchment paper.

2. In a bowl, combine mashed bananas, rolled oats, dark chocolate chips, chopped nuts, cinnamon, and nutmeg (if using).

3. Mix all ingredients until well combined.

4. Using a spoon, drop cookie dough onto the prepared baking sheet, shaping them into cookie rounds.

5. Bake for 12-15 minutes until lightly golden.

6. Allow the cookies to cool on a wire rack before serving.


Greek Yogurt and Berry Parfait

Ingredients:

• Greek yogurt (unsweetened)

• Mixed berries (blueberries, strawberries, raspberries)

• Honey or maple syrup (optional)

• Granola (optional)

Instructions:

1. In serving glasses or bowls, layer Greek yogurt, mixed berries, and a drizzle of honey or maple syrup if desired.

2. Repeat the layers until the glasses are filled.

3. Top with a sprinkle of granola for added crunch if desired.

4. Serve the yogurt and berry parfait immediately.

Apple Cinnamon Baked Oatmeal Cups

Ingredients:

• 2 cups rolled oats

• 2 ripe bananas (mashed)

• 1 cup unsweetened applesauce

• 1/2 cup almond milk (or any milk of choice)

• 1 teaspoon vanilla extract

• 1 teaspoon cinnamon

• 1 apple (diced)

• Chopped nuts (optional)

Instructions:

1. Preheat oven to 350°F (175°C) and grease a muffin tin.

2. In a bowl, mix rolled oats, mashed bananas, applesauce, almond milk, vanilla extract, and cinnamon until combined.

3. Gently fold in diced apples and chopped nuts if using.

4. Spoon the mixture into each muffin cup, filling them to the top. Bake for 25-30 minutes until the tops are golden brown and firm.

5. Let the oatmeal cups cool in the muffin tin before removing and serving.

Avocado Chocolate Mousse

Ingredients:

• 2 ripe avocados

• 1/4 cup unsweetened cocoa powder

• 1/4 cup honey or maple syrup

• 1 teaspoon vanilla extract

• Pinch of salt

• Fresh berries for topping (optional)

Instructions:

1. Scoop out the flesh of ripe avocados and place them in a blender or food processor.

2. Add unsweetened cocoa powder, honey or maple syrup, vanilla extract, and a pinch of salt.

3. Blend until the mixture is smooth and creamy.

4. Transfer the avocado chocolate mousse to serving bowls or glasses.

5. Optionally, top with fresh berries before serving. Refrigerate any leftovers.

Chia Seed Pudding

Ingredients:

• 1/4 cup chia seeds

• 1 cup unsweetened almond milk (or any milk of choice)

• 1 tablespoon honey or maple syrup

• 1/2 teaspoon vanilla extract

• Sliced fruits or nuts for topping (optional)

Instructions:

1. In a bowl, mix chia seeds, unsweetened almond milk, honey or maple syrup, and vanilla extract.

2. Stir well and let the mixture sit for 5 minutes.

3. Stir the mixture again to break up any clumps of chia seeds.

4. Cover the bowl and refrigerate for at least 2 hours or overnight, allowing the chia seeds to absorb the liquid and create a pudding-like consistency.

5. Before serving, stir the pudding and top with sliced fruits or nuts if desired.


Frozen Banana Pops

Ingredients:

• Bananas (peeled and cut in half)

• Greek yogurt (unsweetened)

• Chopped nuts or shredded coconut (optional)

• Wooden popsicle sticks

Instructions:

1. Insert a popsicle stick into each banana half.

2. Dip each banana half into unsweetened Greek yogurt, coating it evenly.

3. Optionally, roll the yogurt-covered banana in chopped nuts or shredded coconut for added texture.

4. Place the coated bananas on a parchment-lined tray and freeze for at least 2 hours until firm.

5. Enjoy these frozen banana pops as a healthy and refreshing dessert.

## Baked Apples with Cinnamon and Walnuts

Ingredients:

• Apples (cored and halved)

• 2 tablespoons chopped walnuts

• 1 tablespoon honey or maple syrup

• 1 teaspoon cinnamon

• Greek yogurt or low-fat whipped cream (optional for serving)

Instructions:

1. Preheat oven to 375°F (190°C).

2. Place cored and halved apples in a baking dish.

3. In a bowl, mix chopped walnuts, honey or maple syrup, and cinnamon. Spoon the mixture into the center of each apple half.

4. Cover the baking dish with foil and bake for 20-25 minutes until apples are tender.

5. Serve the baked apples warm, optionally with a dollop of Greek yogurt or low-fat whipped cream.


Peach and Berry Fruit Salad

Ingredients:

• Peaches (sliced)

• Mixed berries (strawberries, blueberries, raspberries)

• Fresh mint leaves (chopped)

• Honey or a drizzle of balsamic glaze (optional)

Instructions:

1. Combine sliced peaches, mixed berries, and chopped mint leaves in a bowl.

2. Optionally, drizzle honey or balsamic glaze over the fruit salad for added sweetness. Toss gently to coat the fruits.

3. Serve the peach and berry fruit salad immediately.

Almond Butter Energy Bites

Ingredients:

• 1 cup rolled oats

• 1/2 cup almond butter

• 1/4 cup honey or maple syrup

• 1/4 cup unsweetened shredded coconut

• 1/4 cup chopped almonds

• 1 teaspoon vanilla extract

• Pinch of salt

Instructions:

1. In a mixing bowl, combine rolled oats, almond butter, honey or maple syrup, shredded coconut, chopped almonds, vanilla extract, and a pinch of salt.

2. Mix until all ingredients are well combined.

3. Roll the mixture into small bite-sized balls using your hands.

4. Place the energy bites on a plate or baking sheet lined with parchment paper. Refrigerate for at least 30 minutes before serving.

5. Store any leftovers in an airtight container in the refrigerator.

Mango Sorbet

Ingredients:

• 2 ripe mangoes (peeled and chopped)

• 1 tablespoon honey or agave syrup (optional for added sweetness)

• Juice of 1 lime

• Fresh mint leaves for garnish (optional)

Instructions:

1. Place chopped mangoes in a blender or food processor.

2. Add honey or agave syrup (if using) and lime juice. Blend until smooth.

3. Transfer the mango mixture to a shallow dish or ice cube tray. Freeze for 4-6 hours or until set.

4. Before serving, let the sorbet sit at room temperature for a few minutes to soften slightly.

5. Scoop the mango sorbet into serving bowls and garnish with fresh mint leaves if desired.

Yogurt Parfait with Berries and Almonds

Ingredients:

• Greek yogurt (unsweetened)

• Mixed berries (blueberries, raspberries, strawberries)

• Slivered almonds or chopped nuts

• Drizzle of honey or maple syrup (optional)

Instructions:

1. In a glass or bowl, layer Greek yogurt, mixed berries, and slivered almonds.

2. Repeat the layers until the glass is filled.

3. Optionally, drizzle honey or maple syrup over the parfait for added sweetness.

4. Serve the yogurt parfait immediately.

Baked Pears with Cinnamon and Walnuts

Ingredients:

• Pears (halved and cored)

• 1/4 cup chopped walnuts

- 1 tablespoon honey or maple syrup

- 1 teaspoon cinnamon

- Greek yogurt or low-fat whipped cream (optional for serving)

Instructions:

1. Preheat oven to 375°F (190°C).

2. Place halved and cored pears in a baking dish.

3. In a bowl, mix chopped walnuts, honey or maple syrup, and cinnamon. Fill the center of each pear half with the walnut mixture.

4. Cover the baking dish with foil and bake for 20-25 minutes until pears are tender.

5. Serve the baked pears warm, optionally with a dollop of Greek yogurt or low-fat whipped cream.


## Kiwi and Banana Smoothie

Ingredients:

- 2 ripe kiwis (peeled and chopped)

- 1 ripe banana (sliced)

- 1 cup unsweetened almond milk (or any milk of choice)

• Handful of spinach leaves (optional for added nutrients)

• Ice cubes (optional)

• Drizzle of honey or maple syrup (optional for added sweetness)

Instructions:

1. In a blender, combine chopped kiwis, sliced banana, unsweetened almond milk, spinach leaves (if using), and ice cubes if desired.

2. Blend until smooth.

3. Optionally, add a drizzle of honey or maple syrup for added sweetness.

4. Pour the kiwi and banana smoothie into glasses and serve immediately.

Baked Cinnamon Apples

Ingredients:

• 4 apples (cored and sliced)

• 2 tablespoons honey or maple syrup

• 1 teaspoon cinnamon

• 1/4 cup chopped nuts (walnuts or almonds, optional)

• Greek yogurt or low-fat whipped cream (optional for serving)

Instructions:

1. Preheat oven to 375°F (190°C).

2. Place sliced apples in a baking dish. Drizzle honey or maple syrup over the apples.

3. Sprinkle cinnamon and chopped nuts (if using) over the apples. Toss the apples to coat evenly with the mixture.

4. Bake for 20-25 minutes until the apples are tender.

5. Serve the baked cinnamon apples warm, optionally with a dollop of Greek yogurt or low-fat whipped cream.

Blueberry Chia Seed Jam

Ingredients:

• 2 cups fresh blueberries

• 2 tablespoons chia seeds

• 1-2 tablespoons honey or maple syrup (adjust to taste)

• 1 tablespoon lemon juice

Instructions:

1. In a saucepan, heat blueberries over medium heat until they start to break down and release their juices, stirring occasionally.

2. Mash the blueberries with a fork or potato masher to desired consistency.

3. Stir in chia seeds, honey or maple syrup, and lemon juice.

4. Simmer the mixture for 10-15 minutes until it thickens. Remove from heat and let it cool to room temperature.

5. Transfer the blueberry chia seed jam to a jar and refrigerate.

6. Use the jam on toast, yogurt, or as a topping for desserts.


Frozen Yogurt Bark

Ingredients:

• 2 cups Greek yogurt (unsweetened)

• 1/4 cup mixed berries (blueberries, raspberries)

• 2 tablespoons chopped nuts (almonds, pistachios)

• Drizzle of honey or maple syrup (optional for sweetness)

Instructions:

1. Line a baking sheet with parchment paper.

2. Spread Greek yogurt evenly on the parchment paper. Sprinkle mixed berries and chopped nuts over the yogurt.

3. Optionally, drizzle honey or maple syrup over the toppings for added sweetness.

4. Freeze the yogurt bark for at least 3-4 hours until firm.

5. Break the frozen yogurt into pieces before serving.

Orange Granita

Ingredients:

• 2 cups freshly squeezed orange juice

• 1/4 cup honey or agave syrup

• Zest of 1 orange

Instructions:

1. In a bowl, mix freshly squeezed orange juice, honey or agave syrup, and orange zest until well combined.

2. Pour the mixture into a shallow dish or baking pan.

3. Place the dish in the freezer. Every 30 minutes, use a fork to scrape and stir the mixture to create a granita texture.

4. Continue scraping every 30 minutes for about 2-3 hours until the granita is frozen and has a flaky texture.

5. Serve the orange granita in cups or bowls.

Chocolate-Dipped Banana Slices

Ingredients:

• Bananas (peeled and sliced)

• Dark chocolate chips (70% cocoa or higher)

• Chopped nuts or shredded coconut for topping (optional)

Instructions:

1. Line a baking sheet with parchment paper.

2. Insert a toothpick into each banana slice. Melt dark chocolate chips in the microwave in 30-second intervals until smooth.

3. Dip each banana slice into the melted chocolate, coating halfway.

4. Optionally, roll the chocolate-covered part in chopped nuts or shredded coconut.

5. Place the dipped banana slices on the prepared baking sheet and freeze for 20-30 minutes until the chocolate hardens.

Raspberry Chia Seed Popsicles

Ingredients:

• 2 cups fresh raspberries

• 2 tablespoons chia seeds

• 1-2 tablespoons honey or maple syrup (optional for added sweetness)

• 1 cup water

Instructions:

1. In a blender, combine fresh raspberries and water. Blend until smooth.

2. Pour the raspberry mixture into a bowl and stir in chia seeds and honey or maple syrup (if using).

3. Let the mixture sit for 10-15 minutes to allow the chia seeds to swell. Stir the mixture again, then pour it into popsicle molds.

4. Insert popsicle sticks and freeze for at least 4-6 hours until firm.

5. Run the molds under warm water to release the popsicles before serving.


Pineapple Coconut Nice Cream

Ingredients:

- 2 cups frozen pineapple chunks

- 1 ripe banana (frozen)

- 1/2 cup coconut milk (unsweetened)

- Unsweetened shredded coconut for topping (optional)

Instructions:

1. In a food processor or blender, combine frozen pineapple chunks, frozen banana, and coconut milk.

2. Blend until smooth and creamy, scraping down the sides as needed.

3. Transfer the nice cream to a bowl and sprinkle with shredded coconut if desired.

4. Serve immediately as a refreshing dessert.

Dark Chocolate Covered Almonds

Ingredients:

• 1 cup raw almonds

• 4 oz dark chocolate (70% cocoa or higher)

Instructions:

1. Line a baking sheet with parchment paper.

2. In a microwave-safe bowl, melt dark chocolate in 30-second intervals, stirring until smooth.

3. Dip each almond into the melted chocolate, coating it completely.

4. Place the chocolate-covered almonds on the prepared baking sheet. Let them set in the refrigerator for about 20-30 minutes until the chocolate hardens.

5. Enjoy these dark chocolate covered almonds as a delightful snack or dessert.

# Mango Coconut Chia Pudding

Ingredients:

- 1 ripe mango (peeled and chopped)

- 1 cup unsweetened coconut milk

- 1/4 cup chia seeds

- 1 tablespoon honey or maple syrup (optional for sweetness)

- Unsweetened shredded coconut for garnish (optional)

Instructions:

1. Blend the chopped mango and coconut milk in a blender until smooth.

2. Pour the mango-coconut mixture into a bowl and stir in chia seeds and honey or maple syrup (if using).

3. Let the mixture sit for 10-15 minutes, then stir again to prevent clumping.

4. Cover the bowl and refrigerate for at least 2 hours or overnight until the chia seeds absorb the liquid and form a pudding-like consistency.

5. Before serving, sprinkle with unsweetened shredded coconut for garnish if desired.

# Watermelon Lime Granita

Ingredients:

- 4 cups seedless watermelon (cubed)

- Juice of 2 limes

- Zest of 1 lime

- 2 tablespoons honey or agave syrup (optional for sweetness)

Instructions:

1. In a blender, blend watermelon cubes, lime juice, lime zest, and honey or agave syrup (if using) until smooth.

2. Pour the mixture into a shallow dish or baking pan.

3. Place it in the freezer and scrape the mixture with a fork every 30 minutes for about 2-3 hours until it forms a granita-like texture.

4. Serve the watermelon lime granita in cups or bowls.

Green Tea Citrus Cooler

Ingredients:

- 2 green tea bags

- 4 cups water

- Juice of 1 lemon

- Juice of 1 orange

- Fresh mint leaves (optional)

- Ice cubes

Instructions:

1. Boil 4 cups of water and steep green tea bags for 3-5 minutes. Allow the tea to cool to room temperature.

2. In a pitcher, combine the cooled green tea with freshly squeezed lemon and orange juice.

3. Add fresh mint leaves for extra flavor if desired. Refrigerate until chilled.

4. Serve over ice for a refreshing green tea citrus cooler.

Berry and Spinach Smoothie

Ingredients:

* 1 cup fresh spinach leaves

* 1/2 cup mixed berries (blueberries, strawberries, raspberries)

* 1 ripe banana

* 1 cup unsweetened almond milk (or any milk of choice)

* 1 tablespoon chia seeds (optional)

* Ice cubes (optional)

Instructions:

1. In a blender, combine fresh spinach, mixed berries, banana, almond milk, and chia seeds.

2. Blend until smooth and creamy. Add ice cubes for a colder beverage.

3. Pour into glasses and enjoy this nutrient-packed berry and spinach smoothie.

## Cucumber Mint Infused Water

Ingredients:

• 1 cucumber (sliced)

• Handful of fresh mint leaves

• 8 cups water

• Ice cubes

Instructions:

1. In a pitcher, combine sliced cucumber, fresh mint leaves, and water.

2. Refrigerate for at least 2 hours or overnight to infuse the flavors.

3. Serve the refreshing cucumber mint infused water over ice.


## Hibiscus Iced Tea

Ingredients:

• 4 cups water

• 3-4 hibiscus tea bags

• 1-2 tablespoons honey or agave syrup (optional for sweetness)

• Sliced lemon or orange for garnish (optional)

• Ice cubes

Instructions:

1. Bring 4 cups of water to a boil and steep hibiscus tea bags for 5-7 minutes.

2. Remove the tea bags and let the tea cool to room temperature.

3. Optionally, stir in honey or agave syrup for sweetness. Refrigerate until chilled.

4. Serve over ice with sliced lemon or orange for a flavorful iced tea.


Turmeric Golden Milk

Ingredients:

• 2 cups unsweetened almond milk (or any milk of choice)

• 1 teaspoon ground turmeric

• 1/2 teaspoon ground cinnamon

• 1/4 teaspoon ground ginger

• Pinch of black pepper

• 1 tablespoon honey or maple syrup (optional for sweetness)

Instructions:

1. In a small saucepan, warm the almond milk over medium heat.

2. Add ground turmeric, cinnamon, ginger, and a pinch of black pepper. Stir well and simmer for 3-5 minutes without boiling.

3. Optionally, sweeten with honey or maple syrup.

4. Pour into mugs and enjoy this comforting turmeric golden milk.


Mixed Berry Iced Green Tea

Ingredients:

• 2 green tea bags

• 4 cups water

• 1/2 cup mixed berries (blueberries, raspberries, strawberries)

• Fresh mint leaves (optional)

• Ice cubes

Instructions:

1. Boil 4 cups of water and steep green tea bags for 3-5 minutes. Allow the tea to cool to room temperature.

2. In a blender, blend the mixed berries until smooth.

3. In a pitcher, combine the cooled green tea and blended berries. Add fresh mint leaves for extra flavor if desired.

4. Refrigerate until chilled.

5. Serve over ice for a refreshing mixed berry iced green tea.

## Watermelon Basil Cooler

Ingredients:

• 4 cups diced seedless watermelon

• 1/4 cup fresh basil leaves

• Juice of 1 lime

• 4 cups cold water

• Ice cubes

Instructions:

1. In a blender, blend diced watermelon and fresh basil until smooth.

2. Strain the watermelon-basil mixture through a fine-mesh sieve into a pitcher to remove pulp.

3. Add lime juice and cold water to the pitcher and stir well. Refrigerate until chilled.

4. Serve over ice for a refreshing watermelon basil cooler.


Pineapple Ginger Turmeric Smoothie

Ingredients:

• 1 cup fresh pineapple chunks

• 1 banana

• 1/2 teaspoon grated fresh ginger

• 1/4 teaspoon ground turmeric

• 1 cup unsweetened coconut water or almond milk

• Ice cubes

Instructions:

1. In a blender, combine fresh pineapple chunks, banana, grated ginger, ground turmeric, and coconut water or almond milk.

2. Blend until smooth.

3. Add ice cubes for a colder beverage.

4. Pour into glasses and enjoy this pineapple ginger turmeric smoothie.


Minty Lemonade

Ingredients:

• 4 cups water

• Juice of 4-5 lemons

• 1/4 cup fresh mint leaves

• 1/4 cup honey or agave syrup

• Sliced lemon for garnish (optional)

• Ice cubes

Instructions:

1. In a saucepan, bring water to a boil.

2. Add fresh mint leaves and let it steep for 5 minutes. Remove from heat.

3. Strain the mint-infused water into a pitcher. Stir in lemon juice and honey or agave syrup until well combined.

4. Refrigerate until chilled. Serve over ice with a slice of lemon for garnish if desired.


Beet Carrot Apple Juice

Ingredients:

• 2 medium-sized beets (peeled and chopped)

• 2 medium carrots (peeled and chopped)

• 2 apples (cored and chopped)

• 1-inch piece of fresh ginger (peeled)

• Juice of 1 lemon

• Water (as needed for consistency)

• Ice cubes

Instructions:

1. In a juicer, juice the beets, carrots, apples, and ginger.

2. Add the lemon juice to the freshly extracted juice and stir well. Add water to adjust the consistency if desired.

3. Pour the beet carrot apple juice into glasses over ice cubes for a refreshing beverage.

Mango Turmeric Smoothie

Ingredients:

• 1 cup frozen mango chunks

• 1 ripe banana

• 1/2 teaspoon ground turmeric

• 1/2 cup Greek yogurt (unsweetened)

• 1 tablespoon honey or maple syrup (optional for sweetness)

• 1 cup unsweetened almond milk (or any milk of choice)

• Ice cubes

Instructions:

1. In a blender, combine frozen mango chunks, banana, ground turmeric, Greek yogurt, honey or maple syrup (if using), and almond milk.

2. Blend until smooth and creamy. Add ice cubes if desired for a colder beverage.

3. Pour into glasses and enjoy this mango turmeric smoothie.

Herbal Hibiscus Tea

Ingredients:

• 4 cups water

• 3-4 hibiscus tea bags

• 1 tablespoon honey or agave syrup (optional for sweetness)

• Sliced oranges or lemons for garnish (optional)

• Ice cubes

Instructions:

1. Bring 4 cups of water to a boil and steep hibiscus tea bags for 5-7 minutes.

2. Remove the tea bags and let the tea cool to room temperature.

3. Optionally, add honey or agave syrup for sweetness and stir well. Refrigerate until chilled.

4. Serve over ice with slices of oranges or lemons for garnish.

Ingredients:

- 2 cups kale leaves (stems removed)

- 1 cup fresh pineapple chunks

- 1 cucumber (peeled and chopped)

- 1-inch piece of fresh ginger (peeled)

- Juice of 1 lemon

- Ice cubes

Instructions:

1. In a juicer, juice the kale leaves, pineapple chunks, cucumber, and ginger.

2. Add lemon juice to the freshly extracted juice and stir well.

3. Pour the kale pineapple green juice into glasses over ice cubes for a refreshing drink.

Berry-Lemon Infused Water

Ingredients:

• Handful of mixed berries (strawberries, blueberries, raspberries)

• Slices of lemon

• 8 cups water

• Ice cubes

Instructions:

1. In a pitcher, combine mixed berries and slices of lemon. Fill the pitcher with 8 cups of water.

2. Refrigerate for at least 2 hours or overnight to infuse the flavors.

3. Serve the berry-lemon infused water over ice cubes.


Green Apple Mint Sparkler

Ingredients:

• 2 green apples (cored and sliced)

• Fresh mint leaves

• Sparkling water

• Ice cubes

Instructions:

1. In a blender, blend green apple slices and fresh mint leaves until smooth.

2. Strain the blended mixture through a fine-mesh sieve into a pitcher to remove pulp.

3. Fill glasses with ice cubes and pour the strained apple-mint mixture halfway.

4. Top each glass with sparkling water for a fizzy and refreshing green apple mint sparkler.


Carrot Orange Ginger Juice

Ingredients:

• 4 medium carrots (peeled and chopped)

• 2 oranges (peeled and segmented)

• 1-inch piece of fresh ginger (peeled)

• Ice cubes

Instructions:

1. In a juicer, juice the carrots, oranges, and ginger.

2. Stir the juice well to combine flavors.

3. Pour into glasses over ice cubes and serve this refreshing carrot orange ginger juice.

Lemon Basil Infused Water

Ingredients:

• Slices of lemon

• Fresh basil leaves

• 8 cups water

• Ice cubes

Instructions:

1. In a pitcher, combine slices of lemon and fresh basil leaves.

2. Fill the pitcher with 8 cups of water. Refrigerate for at least 2 hours or overnight to infuse the flavors.

3. Serve the lemon basil infused water over ice cubes.

Kiwi Spinach Green Smoothie

Ingredients:

• 2 kiwis (peeled and chopped)

• Handful of fresh spinach leaves

• 1 banana

• 1 cup unsweetened almond milk (or any milk of choice)

• Ice cubes

Instructions:

1. In a blender, combine chopped kiwis, fresh spinach leaves, banana, and almond milk.

2. Blend until smooth. Add ice cubes for a colder beverage.

3. Pour into glasses and enjoy this nutritious kiwi spinach green smoothie.


Minty Watermelon Cooler

Ingredients:

• 4 cups diced seedless watermelon

• Fresh mint leaves

- Juice of 2 limes

- 4 cups cold water

- Ice cubes

Instructions:

1. In a blender, blend diced watermelon and fresh mint leaves until smooth.

2. Strain the watermelon-mint mixture through a fine-mesh sieve into a pitcher to remove pulp.

3. Add lime juice and cold water to the pitcher and stir well.

4. Refrigerate until chilled.

5. Serve over ice for a refreshing minty watermelon cooler.


## Raspberry Cucumber Lemonade

Ingredients:

- 1 cup fresh raspberries

- 1 cucumber (peeled and chopped)

- Juice of 3-4 lemons

- 4 cups cold water

• Ice cubes

Instructions:

1. In a blender, blend fresh raspberries and chopped cucumber until smooth.

2. Strain the raspberry-cucumber mixture through a fine-mesh sieve into a pitcher to remove seeds and pulp.

3. Add lemon juice and cold water to the pitcher and stir well.

4. Refrigerate until chilled.

5. Serve over ice for a refreshing raspberry cucumber lemonade.


## Strawberry Basil Lemonade

Ingredients:

• 2 cups fresh strawberries (hulled)

• Handful of fresh basil leaves

• Juice of 3-4 lemons

• 4 cups cold water

• Ice cubes

Instructions:

1. In a blender, blend fresh strawberries and basil until smooth.

2. Strain the strawberry-basil mixture through a fine-mesh sieve into a pitcher to remove pulp.

3. Add lemon juice and cold water to the pitcher and stir well. Refrigerate until chilled.

4. Serve over ice for a refreshing strawberry basil lemonade.

Blueberry Mint Sparkling Water

Ingredients:

- 1 cup fresh blueberries

- Fresh mint leaves

- Sparkling water

- Ice cubes

Instructions:

1. In a glass or pitcher, muddle fresh blueberries and mint leaves.

2. Fill glasses with ice cubes.

3. Pour the muddled mixture into glasses and top with sparkling water for a fizzy blueberry mint drink.


Pineapple Kale Smoothie

Ingredients:

• 1 cup fresh pineapple chunks

• Handful of kale leaves (stems removed)

• 1 ripe banana

• 1 cup unsweetened coconut water or almond milk

• Ice cubes

Instructions:

1. In a blender, combine pineapple chunks, kale leaves, banana, and coconut water or almond milk.

2. Blend until smooth and creamy. Add ice cubes for a colder beverage.

3. Pour into glasses and enjoy this pineapple kale smoothie.

Ginger-Lemon Turmeric Tea

Ingredients:

• 4 cups water

• 1-inch piece of fresh ginger (peeled and sliced)

• Juice of 2 lemons

• 1/2 teaspoon ground turmeric

• Honey or agave syrup (optional for sweetness)

Instructions:

1. In a saucepan, bring water to a boil and add sliced ginger. Simmer for 10-15 minutes.

2. Remove from heat and strain the ginger-infused water into a pitcher.

3. Add lemon juice, ground turmeric, and sweeten with honey or agave syrup if desired.

4. Stir well and serve this soothing ginger-lemon turmeric tea.

Mango Basil Iced Tea

Ingredients:

- 4 cups water

- 2 black tea bags

- 1 ripe mango (peeled and chopped)

- Handful of fresh basil leaves

- Ice cubes

Instructions:

1. Boil 4 cups of water and steep black tea bags for 3-5 minutes. Allow the tea to cool to room temperature.

2. In a blender, blend chopped mango and basil until smooth.

3. Strain the mango-basil mixture through a fine-mesh sieve into a pitcher to remove pulp.

4. Add the cooled black tea to the pitcher and stir well. Refrigerate until chilled.

5. Serve over ice for a flavorful mango basil iced tea.

# CONCLUSION

In conclusion, adopting the MIND diet can be a transformative step toward enhancing heart health and overall well-being. This dietary approach, crafted from a fusion of the Mediterranean and DASH diets, emphasizes the consumption of brain-boosting and heart-protective foods. By integrating nutrient-rich elements like leafy greens, berries, nuts, whole grains, and lean proteins, the MIND diet not only supports cognitive function but also plays a pivotal role in fortifying cardiovascular health.

Research has shown that adhering to the MIND diet significantly reduces the risk of heart disease by mitigating inflammation, lowering cholesterol levels, regulating blood pressure, and supporting optimal cardiovascular function. This dietary pattern, rich in antioxidants, vitamins, minerals, and healthy fats, offers a powerhouse of nutrients that actively work to combat free radicals and support heart vitality.

The MIND diet doesn't just stop at nourishing the body with beneficial foods; it encompasses a holistic approach to heart health by encouraging a lifestyle centered around mindful eating, regular physical activity, stress management, and quality sleep. By embracing this dietary lifestyle, individuals not only protect their heart but also promote overall health and longevity.

Ultimately, the MIND diet stands as a testament to the profound impact that wholesome and balanced nutrition can have on heart health. Its sustainable approach, grounded in scientific evidence and a wealth of health benefits, offers a pathway to cultivating a healthier heart and a more vibrant life. Embracing the principles of the MIND diet empowers individuals to make mindful choices, savor delicious and nourishing meals, and embark on a journey towards a healthier heart and a brighter future.

www.ingramcontent.com/pod-product-compliance
Lightning Source LLC
Chambersburg PA
CBHW050806260726
48660CB00004B/1281